A PHARMACIST'S GUIDE TO POINT-OF-CARE TESTING

Kristin Wiisanen, PharmD, FAPhA, FCCP
Dean | College of Pharmacy
Rosalind Franklin University of Medicine and Science
North Chicago, Illinois

Jean-Venable "Kelly" R. Goode, PharmD, BCPS, FAPhA, FCCP
Professor and Director, Community-Based Residency Program
Virginia Commonwealth University School of Pharmacy
Richmond, Virginia

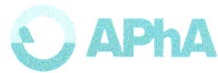

American Pharmacists Association
Washington, D.C.

Senior Director, Books and Digital Publishing: **Eleanore Tapscott**
Editorial Director: **Jesse Vineyard**
Editorial Services: **Michelle Cathers**
Cover: **Kate Erdmann**
Graphic Designer: **Michelle Powell**

©2025 by the American Pharmacists Association
APhA was founded in 1852 as the American Pharmaceutical Association.

Published by the American Pharmacists Association
2215 Constitution Avenue, NW
Washington, DC 20037-2985
www.pharmacist.com
www.pharmacylibrary.com

All rights reserved

No part of this publication may be reproduced, stored in a retrieval system, or transmitted in any form or by any means, electronic, mechanical, photocopying, recording, or otherwise, without written permission from the publisher.

To comment on this book by e-mail, send your message to the publisher at **aphabooks@aphanet.org**.

Library of Congress Cataloging-in-Publication Data available upon request.

How to Order This Book
Online: www.pharmacist.com/shop

NOTICE

The authors, editors, and publisher have made every effort to ensure the accuracy and completeness of the information presented in this book. However, the authors, editors, and publisher cannot be held responsible for the continued currency of the information, any inadvertent errors or omissions, or the application of this information. Therefore, the authors, editors, and publisher shall have no liability to any person or entity with regard to claims, loss, or damage caused or alleged to be caused, directly or indirectly, by the use of information contained herein.

The inclusion in this book of any product in respect to which patent or trademark rights may exist shall not be deemed, and is not intended as, a grant of or authority to exercise any right or privilege protected by such patent or trademark. All such rights or trademarks are vested in the patent or trademark owner, and no other person may exercise the same without express permission, authority, or license secured from such patent or trademark owner.

The inclusion of a brand name does not mean the authors, the editors, or the publisher has any particular knowledge that the brand listed has properties different from other brands of the same product, nor should its inclusion be interpreted as an endorsement by the authors, the editors, or the publisher. Similarly, the fact that a particular brand has not been included does not indicate the product has been judged to be in any way unsatisfactory or unacceptable. Further, no official support or endorsement of this book by any federal or state agency or pharmaceutical company is intended or inferred.

Contributors

Content Coordinator
Emely McKitrick, MPH
Director of Lifelong Learning
University of Florida College of Pharmacy
Gainesville, Florida

Authors

Lindsey M. Childs-Kean, PharmD, MPH, BCPS
Clinical Associate Professor
University of Florida College of Pharmacy
Gainesville, Florida

Stacey D. Curtis, BPharm, PharmD, CPh
Clinical Associate Professor, Assistant Dean for Experiential Education
University of Florida College of Pharmacy
Gainesville, Florida

Sharon Gatewood, PharmD, BCACP, FAPhA
Associate Professor
Virginia Commonwealth University
Richmond, Virginia

Jeffrey Hamper, PharmD, BCACP
Manager, Pharmacy Experiential, Intern, and Residency Programs
Albertsons Companies
Boise, Idaho

Michael Hegener, PharmD, BCACP
Associate Professor, Director – Wuest Family Pharmacy Practice Skills Center
University of Cincinnati James L. Winkle College of Pharmacy
Cincinnati, Ohio

Katelyn Johnson, PharmD, MS, BCACP
Associate Professor
University of Cincinnati James L. Winkle College of Pharmacy
Cincinnati, Ohio

Clark Kebodeaux, PharmD, BCACP
Clinical Associate Professor
University of Kentucky College of Pharmacy
Lexington, Kentucky

Alexis Page, PharmD, BCACP
Deputy Director, Division of Pharmacy Services
Virginia Department of Health
Richmond, Virginia

Traci M. Poole, PharmD, BCACP, BCGP
Associate Professor, Director of Community Practice Advancement
Belmont University
Nashville, Tennessee

Teresa E. Roane, PharmD, MBA, BCACP, CPh
Director, Continuing Pharmacy Education
Co-director, Clinical Pharmacogenomics & Precision Medicine Graduate Program
Director, MTM Professional Certificate Program
Clinical Associate Professor
University of Florida College of Pharmacy
Gainesville, Florida

Rachel Shaddock, PharmD
Clinical Pharmacist, Adjunct Professor
University of Florida College of Pharmacy
Gainesville, Florida

Barbara A. Santevecchi, PharmD, BCIDP
Clinical Assistant Professor
University of Florida College of Pharmacy
Gainesville, Florida

Megan G. Smith, PharmD, BCACP
Associate Professor
University of Arkansas for Medical Sciences
Little Rock, Arkansas

Deanna Tran, PharmD, BCACP, FAPhA
Associate Professor
University of Maryland School of Pharmacy
Baltimore, Maryland

Angelina Vascimini, PharmD, BCACP
Clinical Assistant Professor
University of Florida College of Pharmacy
Gainesville, Florida

Bradley Van Riper, PharmD
Clinical Pharmacy Specialist
UF Health Shands Specialty Pharmacy
Gainesville, Florida

Reviewers

Kenneth C. Hohmeier, PharmD
Professor, Director of Community Affairs, Director of PGY-1 Community-based Pharmacy Residency Program
Health Science Center
The University of Tennessee
Nashville, Tennessee

Fredrica Suarez, PharmD
Pharmacist
Mercyhealth Wisconsin and Illinois
Elgin, Illinois

Table of Contents

SECTION 1: Overview and Implementation of Pharmacy-Based Point-of-Care Testing

- **Chapter 1:** Overview of Point-of-Care Testing and the Role of the Pharmacist 1
- **Chapter 2:** A Stepwise Approach for Developing a Pharmacy-Based CLIA-Waived Laboratory 11
- **Chapter 3:** Point of Care Testing Protocol Development and Requirements 21
- **Chapter 4:** Building a Sustainable Business Model for Point-of-Care Testing Services 33

SECTION 2: Patient Care Through Point-of-Care Testing and Treatment

- **Chapter 5:** Patient Assessment and Point-of-Care Testing 45
- **Chapter 6:** Influenza 59
- **Chapter 7:** Streptococcal Infection 77
- **Chapter 8:** COVID-19 89
- **Chapter 9:** Human Immunodeficiency Virus 101
- **Chapter 10:** Other Disorders Related to Infectious Diseases 113
- **Chapter 11:** Diabetes 133
- **Chapter 12:** Dyslipidemia and Liver Function Abnormalities 143

SECTION 1
Overview and Implementation of Pharmacy-Based Point-of-Care Testing

Overview of Point-of-Care Testing and the Role of the Pharmacist

Rachel Shaddock, PharmD

Key Points

- Stressors to the health care system, including physician shortages, an aging population, and a global pandemic, have expedited the expansion of the role of pharmacists in the health care team.
- Pharmacists are among the most accessible health care professionals in the community setting, as patients visit their community pharmacist about 12 times more frequently than they do their primary care provider.
- There is an opportunity to leverage pharmacists' expertise and unparalleled availability to combat the effects of physician shortages and provide increased access to health care.
- Few states include explicit legislation related to pharmacist's ability to provide point-of-care testing; however, policy interest in pharmacist prescribing has increased.
- Pharmacy-based point-of-care testing services reduce unnecessary antibiotic prescriptions, shorten time from symptom onset to the first dose of treatment, and improve patient satisfaction.

Introduction

Pharmacists have long been charged with the responsibility to use their knowledge and expertise to serve others. When a pharmacist takes the Oath of a Pharmacist, they vow to embrace changes that improve patient care, improve their own professional knowledge, and assure optimal outcomes for all patients.[1] The ways in which pharmacists adhere to this vow have changed greatly over time, but the underlying theme remains the same: to provide the highest quality of patient care to all of those in need.

Since the Oath of a Pharmacist was written, pharmacists' patient care services and pharmacy education efforts have expanded, and they will undoubtedly continue to do so. Stressors to the health care system, including physician shortages, an aging population, and a global pandemic, have helped expedite the expansion of the role of pharmacists in the health care team.[2,3]

Pharmacists who were once viewed as an ancillary member of the team with only the limited role of dispensing medications to their "customers" are now taking on more patient care responsibilities for their "patients" including immunizations, chronic disease management, and point-of-care testing (POCT) with prescriptive authority for minor non-chronic health conditions.[4] State law governs a pharmacist's scope of practice and patient care services, and the extent of prescriptive authority varies state-to-state.[5,6] Descriptions of various types of pharmacist prescriptive authority can be found in Table 1–1. More information about the requirements of protocols is available in Chapter 3. Nevertheless, the general trend continues to be toward increasing patient's access to care by allowing pharmacists to assume more responsibilities as part of an interprofessional health care effort. The focus of this chapter is to identify opportunities to use POCT to test and treat minor health conditions under an established protocol in the pharmacy setting while highlighting the positive impact of POCT on patient care and satisfaction.

Table 1–1. Prescriptive authority definitions

Term	Definition
Collaborative practice agreement (CPA)	Pharmacist prescriptive authority strategy in which pharmacists can initiate and modify selected prescription medications for both chronic and non-chronic conditions, as outlined in a protocol, under the supervision of a physician who also cares for the patient (e.g., collaborative hypertension management)[3,15] The CPA may be patient-specific, population-specific, or medication-specific.[5,6]
Government protocol	Pharmacist prescriptive authority strategy in which pharmacists can prescribe a medication for patients following a protocol that specifies pharmacist training, specified patient inclusion and exclusion criteria, and specific medications, in a non-patient-specific protocol (e.g., statewide protocol for naloxone).[3,15] Protocols may be local, state, or federal.[5]
Standard-of-care prescribing	This type of prescribing is similar to physician prescribing. Pharmacists use their own professional judgment to prescribe medications within a standard of care, that is, what other prudent pharmacists would do in the same or similar situation.[5] For pharmacists, prescribing may require or not require a diagnosis.[5]
Dependent prescribing	Pharmacist prescribing pursuant to a collaborative practice agreement.[5]
Independent prescribing	Pharmacists independently prescribe certain drugs in certain circumstances, either through a government protocol or through standard-of-care prescribing.[5]

Evolution of Point-of-Care Technology

POCT is diagnostic testing that takes place near the patient's site of care outside of a clinical laboratory with the use of a portable device.[4,7] These tests obtain rapid and real-time results to allow caregivers to make patient care decisions within minutes. POCT has been used for years to monitor chronic disease states in a doctor's office (cholesterol panels, glycated hemoglobin, and international normalized ratio [INR]), as well as to monitor acute conditions at the patient's bedside, including electrolyte abnormalities and infectious diseases.[7] Pharmacists have used POCT for decades to screen patients for disease and monitor drug therapy by conducting testing similar to that used in physician practices.[8,9] POCT also provides opportunities for rapid diagnostic testing to quickly diagnose infectious diseases. POCT tests fall under the Clinical Laboratory Improvements Amendments 1988 (CLIA) and most are considered waived tests.[10] The types of test categories are waived, moderately complex, and highly complex; waived tests are simple to conduct, with minimal risk of error, whereas moderately complex and highly complex tests require more training or testing experience and more frequent quality control.[11] As POCT technology advanced, testing devices became easier to use and more portable, allowing for POCT to be used by individuals with minimal training in various practice sites, including pharmacies and patient's homes.[7]

Test-and-treat initiatives take the concept of POCT further by providing treatment recommendations in real-time based on the results of testing to screen and diagnose patients at increased risk for a particular condition.[12] Historically, test-and-treat initiatives have been population-based strategies.[12] Pharmacists have adopted the test-and-treat term to refer to the use of POCT (testing) and prescription of treatment (treat) as a result of patient presentation and testing. At the legislative level, the use of test-and-treat language expands the responsibility for diagnosis and prescribing treatments from physicians to include other health professions, thus modernizing the scope of pharmacist practice; however, this shift has been controversial. Table 1–2 summarizes definitions related to this topic. Pharmacists' authority to provide test-and-treat services, protocol requirements, and disease states

Table 1–2. Testing definitions

Term	Definition
Point-of-care testing (POCT)	Diagnostic testing that takes place near the patient's site of care outside of a clinical laboratory with the use of a CLIA-waived device.[4,5]
Rapid diagnostic test (RDT)	Group of tests designed to detect pathogen-specific antigens, nucleic acid sequences, or host antibody responses to certain pathogens with short performance times, and may be performed under a certificate of waiver.[40]
Test-and-treat (TNT)	Intervention strategy in which a population is screened for a disease state/condition using POCT and treatment is prescribed for eligible patients based on test results.[12]
Clinical Laboratory Improvement Amendments of 1988 (CLIA)	Regulations are comprised of federal standards that apply to all U.S. facilities that test specimens collected from a human being for health assessment or to diagnose, prevent, or treat humans.[10,11]

covered as part of these services vary by state. However, the use of test-and-treat specifically in the pharmacy setting to detect, triage, and provide treatment for various acute conditions such as influenza or streptococcal pharyngitis has gained traction as pharmacies have become a destination for patients to seek medical advice, unloading some of the strain on urgent care settings and emergency departments.[2] In March 2022, the Biden-Harris Administration introduced a nationwide Test to Treat initiative to increase access to affordable COVID-19 treatment, allowing pharmacists to conduct POCT services for COVID-19 and prescribe treatment to those who meet certain requirements regardless of current state legislation, which increased awareness and public perception.[13]

Overview of the Health System and Pharmacists' Unique Position

National organizations such as the Centers for Disease Control and Prevention (CDC) and the U.S. Department of Health and Human Services (HHS) have envisioned the need for health care reform to improve access to care and reduce health disparities.[14,15] The focus on increasing access to care is in part due to both current and projected physician shortages, as well as the strain on the health care system due to COVID-19.[2,16] The Association of American Medical Colleges (AAMC) reports a projected total physician shortage of between 37,800 and 124,000 physicians by the year 2034.[17] The workforce shortage problems are especially apparent in the primary care setting and in rural areas. The patient-to-primary care physician ratio in rural areas is 39.8 physicians per 100,000 people, while the ratio in urban areas is 53.5 physicians per 100,000 people.[18] These shortages reveal a workload that is not sustainable as the population continues to age and highlight the importance of using a team of health care providers, including pharmacists, to provide quality patient care.[3]

Because pharmacists are often recognized as one of the most accessible health care professionals in community-based settings, there is an opportunity to leverage pharmacists' expertise and unparalleled availability to combat the effects of physician shortages and provide increased access to health care. Pharmacies are located throughout the community and often can be reached while grocery shopping or via a drive-thru, as well as after work and on weekends. About 90% of Americans live within 5 miles of a pharmacy, and patients visit their community pharmacist about 12 times more frequently than they do their primary care provider.[19,20] Therefore, pharmacists are uniquely positioned to offer testing and treatment to communities using POCT and prescriptive authority, eliminating access as a barrier to receiving care.[16]

Current Landscape

The lack of access to quality and timely health care often leaves patients with limited choices when facing an acute health condition. By providing POCT to triage these minor conditions, pharmacists create a more resilient health care system and provide additional options for patients to receive necessary care at convenient locations in community-based settings.[16] Allowing pharmacists to prescribe treatments based on the results of POCT via test-and-treat strategies leads to earlier access to care and treatment for patients, which can be lifesaving. Pharmacists can initiate and modify selected prescription medications via dependent prescribing, as well as by collaborative prescribing as established by a collaborative practice agreement (CPA).[3,5] However, these services are not currently offered at every pharmacy and the extent of prescriptive authority varies widely. As alluded to previously, this variation can be explained by the fact that the scope of pharmacy practice is regulated at the state level in the United States.[21]

Independent prescribing allows a pharmacist to prescribe medications for patients that meet specified criteria, and the formulary and amount of medications that can be prescribed are generally limited in comparison with those of physicians.[3,5,21] Two examples of independent prescribing in statewide protocols are birth control medications and naloxone.[21] Dependent and independent prescribing can be used for both chronic and non-chronic conditions, allowing a pharmacist to initiate, modify, or discontinue prescription medications under their state-determined scope of practice or a written agreement or protocol with a supervising physician.[3,5,21] Dependent prescribing under a CPA typically only occurs for patients collaboratively managed by a pharmacist and physician, whereas independent prescribing can be done for any patient in a given state if they meet the outlined requirements of that state.[21] While there are advantages and disadvantages to each prescriptive authority model, the general trend has been toward more legislation specifically allowing pharmacy-based POCT. At this time, few states include explicit legislation related to the ability of pharmacists to provide POCT; however, policy interest in pharmacist prescribing has started to increase.[21,22]

The first steps toward pharmacist prescribing occurred in 1979 in Washington State, when its Pharmacy Practice Act was amended to authorize pharmacists to broadly initiate and modify drug therapy. Although not specific to non-chronic conditions in the setting of POCT, this amendment allowed pharmacists in Washington to provide expanded pharmacy services such as management of medications for asthma and diabetes.[23] To further support pharmacists, Washington also passed state legislation to give pharmacists provider status and allow them to bill for their clinical services.[23] Washington's progressive pursuit of provider status and expanded pharmacy services paved the way for other states. As of the end of 2023, more than 20 states allowed prescribing authority for pharmacists to treat specific health conditions that can be detected via a CLIA-waived diagnostic test under a statewide protocol or as part of a CPA with a supervising physician.[22] Each state varies with regard to the disease states that can be treated; however, the most commonly included disease states tend to require minimal treatment, including influenza, streptococcal pharyngitis, and urinary tract infections (UTIs).[22] Among states that allow test-and-treat services in the pharmacy setting, the prerequisites for pharmacists wishing to offer these services vary widely; important state-to-state differences are highlighted below.

Kentucky legislation allows pharmacists to use board-approved and physician-signed protocols to test and treat for influenza, streptococcal pharyngitis, UTIs, and other self-limiting non-chronic conditions.[22,24] Prior to providing these services, the protocols specify that pharmacists must receive education and training from a provider accredited by the Accreditation Council for Pharmacy Education (ACPE) or approved by the Kentucky Board of Pharmacy. The protocols also contain information regarding inclusion criteria, exclusion criteria, medications that can be prescribed by a pharmacist, and procedures related to follow-up, monitoring, documentation, and physician notification.[24]

In February 2022, Florida passed legislation to allow pharmacists to test and treat patients for minor, non-chronic health conditions that are generally managed with minimal treatment or self-care, including, but not limited to, influenza and streptococcal infections.[25] In order to provide these services, a Florida pharmacist must add a Pharmacist

Test and Treat Certification to their license and complete a 20-hour Florida Board of Pharmacy-approved certification course.[26] Florida also requires pharmacists to enter into a written protocol with a supervising physician outlining the specific categories of patients the pharmacist may treat, physician instructions for patient assessment and treatment for the pharmacist to follow, and a schedule and process for the pharmacist to notify the physician of the treatment plan for each patient.[25,26] These are just two examples of significant advancements on the state level to improve access to care; however, several opportunities exist for further policy breakthroughs.[3] Montana and Idaho have expanded pharmacists' scope of practice related to independent prescribing under a standard-of-care prescribing model, under which pharmacists are granted broad authority to administer, interpret, and act on test results if they have the necessary clinical ability.[5] Montana's model is non-diagnostic, while Idaho has included prescribing within the pharmacist's scope of practice.[5]

Impact of Pharmacy-Based Point-of-Care Testing

The impact of pharmacy-based test-and-treat services has been studied in several countries, including the United Kingdom, Canada, New Zealand, and the United States.[27,28] Aside from the convenience, these services have been shown to reduce unnecessary antibiotic prescriptions, shorten the time from symptom onset to the first dose of treatment, and improve patient satisfaction. In Canada, the RxOUTMAP study analyzing pharmacist-led POCT for UTIs reported that a majority of the participants expressed a high level of trust in their pharmacist, appreciated the accessibility of the pharmacist, and were ultimately very satisfied with their visit.[29]

Acute pharyngitis is generally self-limiting and can be caused by a variety of bacteria and viruses, with viral infection being more common.[30] About 70–95% of pharyngitis cases are caused by viruses, yet about 60% of patients are prescribed antibiotics after presenting with a sore throat.[30,31] Pharmacy-based POCT for *Streptococcus* presents an opportunity to promote prompt access to antibiotic therapy for patients, while preventing severe complications and avoiding unnecessary treatment of patients with viral pharyngitis.[31] An observational study that retrospectively analyzed 204 pharmacy locations in Canada providing POCT for streptococcal pharyngitis found that 68.7% of those who tested positive received an antibiotic prescription within the same day, while only 5.6% of those who tested negative received a same-day antibiotic prescription. A few of the pharmacy locations did not have prescriptive authority, so the antibiotics prescribed to those who tested negative resulted from medical referral. Patients who participated in pharmacy-based POCT were surveyed, and 81% of participants reported that they were either very satisfied or satisfied with the service, while 93% of respondents reported that they would be very likely or somewhat likely to use the service in the future. The most common reasons cited for wanting to use the service again were efficient service (54%) and quick results (26%).[31]

Another disease state with boundless potential for pharmacist impact is influenza. Antiviral treatment for influenza is most effective when taken within 48 hours of symptom onset, making access to timely care of the utmost importance.[32] A multicenter study of 13 pharmacies in four states throughout the United States randomized 27 patients and compared the efficiency of POCT services when pharmacists could prescribe oseltamivir as part of a pre-arranged physician-approved CPA (treatment group) versus POCT services when pharmacists could conduct the testing and had no prescriptive authority, so that patients with a positive result had to be referred to their primary care provider for treatment (referral group). For those who were prescribed oseltamivir, the mean time to the first dose was significantly reduced from 385.3 minutes in the referral group to 57.8 minutes in the treatment group.[33] Although the sample size was small, this study shows that POCT paired with prescriptive authority can shorten the time to treatment for diseases with public health importance such as influenza.

Opportunities in Pharmacy-Based Point-of-Care Testing

POCT and test-and-treat services in a pharmacy setting are not just convenient options for patients; for some patients, they are the only option. Findings from a multicenter study analyzing 55 community pharmacies offering POCT for streptococcal pharyngitis from October 2013 to August 2014 revealed that only a little over 50% of the patients had a primary care provider and more than 40% of the study population accessed the POCT services during evening hours, on the weekends, and on holidays.[34] Furthermore, in 2017, the average wait time between a patient calling a doctor's office and seeing a physician to complete a routine physical was 24 days for a new patient visit and 29 days for an established patient.[3] Therefore, while access to health care services is a major concern, timely access is just as important in ensuring the detection and treatment of non-chronic conditions in patients with limited access to health care providers. Allowing pharmacists to test for these conditions utilizing a test-and-treat strategy can alleviate some of the burden on urgent care centers, emergency departments, and primary care offices to ultimately improve patient outcomes.

In order to provide POCT services, pharmacies must enroll as a CLIA-waived testing location through the Centers for Medicare and Medicaid Services (CMS).[2] The procedures for enrollment include completing the appropriate form, paying biennial fees, and complying with the manufacturer-recommended policies and procedures for each testing device to ensure safe and accurate POCT.[7] As of 2020, approximately 15,671 pharmacy locations were registered as a CLIA-waived testing site, which represents a significant increase from 10,626 CLIA-waived pharmacy testing sites in 2015.[35] It is likely that there are several reasons for this 45% increase in testing sites over a 5-year period, but this change was mainly driven by COVID-19 testing efforts in the pharmacy setting. In addition, the percentage of pharmacies with a CLIA waiver varies significantly by state, with the lowest prevalence (2.92% of pharmacies) in Pennsylvania and the greatest prevalence (56.52% of pharmacies) in Washington.[35]

In addition to the regulatory barriers to implementing pharmacy-based POCT and test-and-treat services, logistical barriers to implementing these services have been addressed in the literature. To demystify the myth that POCT would not be feasible to incorporate into the community pharmacy setting, a time-and-motion study examining three community-based pharmacy locations offering influenza rapid diagnostic testing (RDT) found that the average time to complete a patient encounter, including testing, was 35.5 minutes (± 3.1 minutes), while the average pharmacist participation time per encounter was 9.4 minutes (± 3 minutes). From the patient's perspective, the total average wait time was 20.6 minutes, most of which was due to the time waiting for the RDT result.[36]

Recent national efforts to detect, treat, and prevent human immunodeficiency virus (HIV) in order to dampen its spread created an opportunity for pharmacists to implement HIV POCT services in the pharmacy setting. In 2021, there were more than 1.2 million people living with HIV in the United States, and 13% of those people were unaware of their infection and therefore unlikely to prevent transmission of the disease or obtain appropriate treatment.[37] In the setting of HIV, pharmacies provide a non-stigmatizing and accepting setting that is conducive to providing HIV prevention and treatment strategies in real-time for those at risk.[38] A study conducted in a single independent community pharmacy in Washington analyzed the value of pharmacy-based HIV POCT provided to 50 participants. They found that although POCT only detected 1 HIV patient who tested positive, the pharmacist's assessment led to 76% of the study population (n = 38) qualifying for and receiving preexposure prophylaxis (PrEP) therapy.[39] Pharmacist referrals to an alternative health care provider were made for 28 participants, and 71% of those referred established care with a health care provider following their interaction at the pharmacy.[39] Whether they are initiating antiretroviral therapy or recommending postexposure and preexposure prophylaxis (PEP and PrEP), pharmacists have opportunities to help end the HIV epidemic by providing care to patients who may not have been able to be screened otherwise and linking patients to appropriate health care providers.

Conclusion

From the advent of Medication Therapy Management services and immunization authority to collaborative practice and test-and-treat strategies using POCT, the focus of pharmacists continues to shift from the drug product to the patient. This shift was tested during the coronavirus pandemic, when the HHS authorized all pharmacists to provide COVID-19 testing regardless of state law in order to increase access to care in a time of urgent need.[13,20] The COVID-19 pandemic reaffirmed the importance of pharmacists practicing at the highest level of their license and the need to expand their clinical role to include the ability to test and screen for various minor health conditions. Pharmacists with prescriptive authority to provide treatment for those with a positive result, as well as symptom management and education for those with a negative result was instrumental during the pandemic. In addition, patients continue to report the convenience of quality care as an important factor for determining their preferred site of care.[41] Pharmacists are uniquely positioned to serve as an alternative avenue for patients to receive quality care in a timely manner.

References

1. American Pharmacists Association. Oath of a pharmacist. Available at: https://www.pharmacist.com/About/Oath-of-a-Pharmacist. Accessed March 26, 2023.

2. Zikry G, Bach A. Point-of-care resting offers new opportunities. *Pharmacy Times*. Available at: www.pharmacytimes.com/view/point-of-care-testing-offers-new-opportunities. Accessed February 10, 2024.

3. Sachdev G, Kliethermes MA, Vernon V, et al. Current status of prescriptive authority by pharmacists in the United States. *J Am Coll Clin Pharm.* 2020;3: 807–817. doi:10.1002/jac5.1245

4. Urick BY, Meggs EV. Towards a greater professional standing: Evolution of pharmacy practice and education, 1920–2020. *Pharmacy.* 2019;7(3):98. doi:10.3390/pharmacy7030098

5. Adams A, Weaver KK, Adams JA. Revisiting the continuum of pharmacist prescriptive authority. *J Am Pharm Assoc.* 2023;63:1508–1514. doi:10.1016/j.japh.2023.06.025

6. Centers for Disease Control and Prevention. Collaborative Practice Agreements and Pharmacists' Patient Care Services: A resource for pharmacists. Atlanta, GA: CDC. Available at: https://www.cdc.gov/dhdsp/pubs/docs/translational_tools_pharmacists.pdf . Accessed February 10, 2024.

7. Kehrer JP, James DE. The role of pharmacists and pharmacy education in point-of-care testing. *Am J Pharm Educ.* 2016;80(8):Article 129. doi:10.5688/ajpe808129

8. Bluml BM, McKenney JM, Cziraky MJ, et al. Interim report from project ImPACT: Hyperlipidemia. *J Am Pharm Assoc.* 1998;38:529–534. doi:10.1016/s1086-5802(16)30377-1

9. Cranor CW, Bunting BA, Christensen DB. The Asheville Project: Long-term clinical and economic outcomes of a community pharmacy diabetes care program. *J Am Pharm Assoc.* 2003;43;173–184. doi:10.1331/108658003321480713

10. Centers for Disease Control and Prevention. Clinical Laboratory Improvement Amendments (CLIA). Atlanta, GA: CDC. Available at: https://www.cdc.gov/clia/index.html. Accessed February 10, 2024.

11. U.S. Food and Drug Administration. CLIA Classifications. Silver Spring, MD: FDA. Available at: https://www.fda.gov/medical-devices/ivd-regulatory-assistance/clia-categorizations#:~:text=The%20FDA%20categorizes%20diagnostic%20tests,tests%2C%20and%20high%20complexity%20tests. Accessed February 10, 2024.

12. Nah K, Nishiura H, Tsuchiya N, et al. Test-and-treat approach to HIV/AIDS: A primer for mathematical modeling. *Theor Biol Med Model.* 2017;14:Article 16. doi:10.1186/s12976-017-0062-9

13. U.S. Department of Health and Human Services. Test to Treat. Washington, DC: HHS. Available at: https://aspr.hhs.gov/TestToTreat/Pages/default.aspx. Accessed February 10, 2024.

14. U.S. Department of Health and Human Services. Advancing public health through law and policy. Washington, DC: HHS. Available at: https://health.gov/our-work/national-health-initiatives/healthy-people/healthy-people-2020/healthy-people-2020-law-and-health-policy. Accessed February 10, 2024.

15. Health.gov. Health Care Access and Quality. Healthy People 2030. Available at: https://health.gov/healthy-people/objectives-and-data/browse-objectives/health-care-access-and-quality. Accessed February 10, 2024.

16. Smith DJ, McGill L, Carranza D, et al. Global engagement of pharmacists in test and treat initiatives: Bringing care from clinics to communities. *J Am Pharm Assoc.* 2023;63:419–423. doi:10.1016/j.japh.2022.10.013

17. Association of American Medical Colleges. Markit I. The complexities of physician supply and demand: projections from 2019 to 2034. Available at: https://www.aamc.org/media/54681/download. Accessed February 10, 2024.

18. U.S. Department of Health and Human Services, Centers for Disease Control and Prevention, National Center for Health Statistics. Hing E, Hsiao C. State Variability in Supply of Office-based Primary Care Providers, United States, 2012. No. 2014. Available at: https://www.cdc.gov/nchs/data/databriefs/db151.pdf. Accessed February 10, 2024.

19. Berenbrok LA, Tang S, Gabriel N, et al. Access to community pharmacies: A nationwide geographic information systems cross-sectional analysis. *J Am Pharm Assoc.* 2022;62:1816–1822.e2. doi:10.1016/j.japh.2022.07.003

20. Strand MA, Bratberg JM, Eukel H, et al. Community pharmacists' contributions to disease management during the COVID-19 pandemic. *Prev Chronic Dis.* 2020;17. doi:10.5888/pcd17.200317

21. Page, A, Owen JA, Goode JR, et al. Pharmacist-initiated treatment of minor conditions: A call to action. *J Am Pharm Assoc* 2021;61:13–19. doi:10.1016/j.japh.2020.09.021

22. National Alliance of State Pharmacy Associations. Pharmacist prescribing: "test and treat." Washington, DC: NASPA. Available at: https://naspa.us/resource/pharmacist-prescribing-for-strep-and-flu-test-and-treat. Accessed February 10, 2024.

23. Hazlet TK, Karwaki TE, Downing DF. Pathway to pharmacist medical provider status in Washington State. *J Am Pharm Assoc.* 2017;57:116–119. doi:10.1016/j.japh.2016.09.003

24. Kentucky Board of Pharmacy. Board Approved Protocols. Available at: https://pharmacy.ky.gov/Pages/search.aspx?terms=protocols&affiliateId=-pharmacy.ky.gov. Accessed February 10, 2024.

25. Official Internet Site of the Florida Legislature. The 2022 Florida Statutes. Available at: http://www.leg.state.fl.us/statutes/index.cfm?App_mode=Display_Statute&Search_String=&URL=0400-0499%2F0465%2FSections%2F0465.1895.html. Accessed February 10, 2024.

26. Florida Board of Pharmacy. Pharmacist test and treat certification. Available at: https://floridaspharmacy.gov/licensing/pharmacist-test-and-treat-certification/#tab-requirementseac2-37be. Accessed February 10, 2024.

27. Klepser ME, Adams AJ. Pharmacy-based management of influenza: lessons learned from research. *Int J Pharm Pract*. 2018;26:573–578. doi:10.1111/ijpp.12488

28. Mahoney MV, Bhagat H, Christian R, et al. Pharmacists as important prescribers of coronavirus disease 2019 (COVID-19) antivirals. *Antimicrob Steward Healthc Epidemiol*. 2022;2:e112. doi:10.1017/ash.2022.248

29. Beahm NP, Smyth DJ, Tsuyuki RT. Outcomes of Urinary Tract Infection Management by Pharmacists (RxOUTMAP): A study of pharmacist prescribing and care in patients with uncomplicated urinary tract infections in the community. *Can Pharm J (Ott)*. 2018; 151:305–314. doi:10.1177/1715163518781175

30. Shulman ST, Bisno AL, Clegg HW, et al. Clinical practice guideline for the diagnosis and management of group A streptococcal pharyngitis: 2012 update by the Infectious Diseases Society of America. *Clin Infect Dis*. 2012;55:1279–82. doi:10.1093/cid/cis847

31. Papastergiou J, Trieu CR, Saltmarche D, et al. Community pharmacist–directed point-of-care group A Streptococcus testing: Evaluation of a Canadian program. *J Am Pharm Assoc*. 2018;58:450–456. doi:10.1016/j.japh.2018.03.003

32. Uyeki TM, Bernstein HH, Bradley JS, et al. Clinical practice guidelines by the Infectious Diseases Society of America: 2018 update on diagnosis, treatment, chemoprophylaxis, and institutional outbreak management of seasonal influenza. *Clin Infect Dis*. 2019;68:e1–e47. doi:10.1093/cid/ciy866

33. Klepser ME, Hagerman JK, Klepser SA, et al. A community pharmacy-based influenza screening and management program shortens time to treatment versus pharmacy screening with referral to standard of care. *Ill Pharm*. 2014;76:12–18.

34. Klepser DG, Klepser ME, Dering-Anderson AM, et al. Community pharmacist–physician collaborative streptococcal pharyngitis management program. *J Am Pharm Assoc*. 2016;56:323–329. doi:10.1016/j.japh.2015.11.013

35. Klepser NS, Klepser DG, Adams JL, et al. Impact of COVID-19 on prevalence of community pharmacies as CLIA-waived facilities. *Res Soc Admin Pharm*. 2021;17:1574–1578. doi:10.1016/j.sapharm.2020.12.003

36. Klepser D, Dering-Anderson A, Morse J, et al. Time and motion study of influenza diagnostic testing in a community pharmacy. *Innov Pharm*. 2014;5(2): Article 159. doi:10.24926/iip.v5i2.341

37. Centers for Disease Control and Prevention. HIV Basics. Atlanta, GA: CDC. Available at: https://www.cdc.gov/hiv/basics/statistics.html. Accessed February 10, 2024.

38. McCree DH, Byrd KK, Johnston M, et al. Roles for pharmacists in the "Ending the HIV epidemic: A plan for America" initiative. *Public Health Rep*. 2020; 135:547–554. doi:10.1177/0033354920941184

39. Kherghehpoush S, McKeirnan KC. The role of community pharmacies in the HIV and HCV care continuum. *Explor Res Clin Soc Pharm*. 2023;9:100215. doi:10.1016/j.rcsop.2022.100215

40. Centers for Disease Control and Prevention. Rapid Diagnostic Tests for Infectious Diseases. Atlanta, GA: CDC. Available at: https://wwwnc.cdc.gov/travel/yellowbook/2024/posttravel-evaluation/rapid-diagnostic-tests-for-infectious-diseases. Accessed February 10, 2024.

41. Hohmeier KC, Loomis B, Gatwood J. Consumer perceptions of and willingness-to-pay for point-of-care testing services in the community pharmacy. *Res Soc Admin Pharm*. 2018;14:360–366. doi:10.1016/j.sapharm.2017.04.011

CHAPTER 2

A Stepwise Approach for Developing a Pharmacy-Based CLIA-Waived Laboratory

Stacey D. Curtis, BPharm, PharmD, CPh and
Angelina Vascimini, PharmD, BCACP

Key Points

- Pharmacists may use an 8-step approach for successful development and implementation of a pharmacy-based CLIA-waived laboratory.
- Testing personnel are required to complete a variety of types of training, including training regarding Occupational Safety and Health Administration (OSHA) Bloodborne Pathogen Standards. OSHA outlines standards for this training.
- As the scope of community-based pharmacy practice continues to evolve toward clinical appointment-based models, community pharmacy CLIA-waived laboratory applications are vital for implementing point-of-care testing.

Introduction

Implementing pharmacy-based point-of-care testing (POCT) into a new or already established community pharmacy expands clinical patient care services while simultaneously increasing revenue for the pharmacy. Several steps are required to develop and implement such services, which may seem daunting. However, this chapter serves to provide step-by-step instructions to simplify and streamline the process. Pharmacy practice laws vary by state and should be reviewed prior to starting this process.

Step 1: Preparation

Several items must be considered before offering point-of-care clinical services within a community pharmacy. The initial and most crucial step is to evaluate costs associated with the development and implementation of the services, which include, but are not limited to, time, licenses and fees, equipment and supplies, personnel, record keeping and additional resources. Once costs have been evaluated, the value-added benefits of the clinical services must also be reviewed to calculate how much revenue can be generated based on each clinical service added. While analyzing this information is time-consuming, it allows pharmacy owners to determine what must be done to reap the benefits of implementing point-of-care services.

Step 2: Testing Oversight

Oversight over the laboratory is the responsibility of the laboratory director, whose primary focus should consist of overseeing testing, decision making, and the overall environment of the facility and workspace. It is important to identify an individual to oversee the laboratory and follow good laboratory practices outlined by the Centers for Medicare & Medicaid Services (CMS).[1] Additionally, some essential attributes to consider when hiring the laboratory director include professional attitude, interpersonal communication skills, motivation, organizational skills, focus, problem solving ability, honesty and integrity, manual dexterity, mathematical skills and good eyesight.[2]

Step 3: Regulatory Considerations for Testing

Laboratory quality and safety remain a top priority for all health care institutions. Regulatory and accrediting agencies oversee the development, implementation, and continuation of point-of-care services in community pharmacies. It is important to understand and follow all regulatory requirements.

Clinical Laboratory Improvement Amendments

The Clinical Laboratory Improvement Amendments of 1988 (CLIA) regulations are comprised of federal standards that apply to all United States facilities that test specimens collected from a human being for health assessment or for diagnosis, prevention, or treatment.[3] The U.S. Food and Drug Administration (FDA), Centers for Disease Control and Prevention (CDC), and CMS all work together to implement the CLIA program.[3] Each agency has a specific role (see Table 2–1 for additional information) in assuring laboratory testing quality, with CMS acting as the regulating agency that provides the CLIA Certificate of Waiver.[4] As defined by CLIA, waived tests are "simple laboratory examinations and procedures that have an insignificant risk of an erroneous result."[5] Under CLIA, these low-risk tests can be performed with no routine regulatory oversight.[6]

Table 2–1. Regulating agencies and their roles[16]

Agency	Role
U.S. Food and Drug Administration (FDA)	• Categorizes tests based on complexity • Reviews requests for Waiver by Application • Develops rules/guidance for CLIA complexity categorization
Centers for Disease Control (CDC)	• Providing analysis, research, and technical assistance • Developing technical standards and laboratory practice guidelines, including standards and guidelines for cytology • Conducting laboratory quality improvement studies • Monitoring proficiency testing practices • Developing and distributing professional information and educational resources • Managing the Clinical Laboratory Improvement Advisory Committee (CLIAC)
Centers for Medicare & Medicaid Services (CMS)	• Issues laboratory certificates • Collects user fees • Conducts inspections and enforces regulatory compliance • Approves private accreditation organizations for performing inspections and approves state exemptions • Monitors laboratory performance on PT and approves PT programs • Publishes CLIA rules and regulations

Key: CLIA, Clinical Laboratory Improvement Amendments of 1988; PT, proficiency testing.

Some of the most frequently used CLIA low-risk tests in the community pharmacy setting are listed in Box 2–1.[3] A critical component of adding point-of-care services is the implementation of CLIA-waived tests to increase access for patient care services, with the overall goal of improving public health.

Box 2–1. Common low-risk CLIA-waived tests[3]

- Blood glucose
- Cholesterol panel
- HbA1C
- Hepatitis C testing
- HIV testing
- Influenza testing
- INR
- Sexually transmitted infection tests (chlamydia, gonorrhea, hepatitis, HIV, herpes, syphilis, trichomoniasis, genital warts)
- Streptococcal pharyngitis test
- Urine albumin
- Urine analysis (urinary tract infection testing)
- Urine drug screening

Applying for a CLIA Certificate of Waiver

In order for a pharmacy to develop a pharmacy-based CLIA-waived laboratory eligible to perform POCT and treatment, the facility must enroll in the CLIA program by completing the application (Form CMS-116), which is available on the CMS CLIA website (www.cms.gov/medicare/cms-forms/cms-forms/cms-forms-items/cms012169), and obtain a certificate of waiver.[5] The application assembles all required data necessary as an overview of the facility operations to determine quality and assess fees. The health care provider (HCP) who will serve as the director of the laboratory must provide information in the application, including their name, credentials, and contact information.[5] The application also requires the facility to identify the waived testing to be performed, including each analyte, test system, and device that will be used.[5] A complete list of the currently approved materials, systems, and devices can be found on the FDA website.[4] The completed application shall be sent to the appropriate local state agency in the state in which the facility is located.[5] The requirements of each state may be slightly different; therefore, it is critical to check for state-specific requirements.[5] It is also important to note that each individual site where testing will be done must complete a separate application.[5] In addition, if a site decides to add an additional test, they must notify CMS. If online access and/or information from the appropriate state agency is not available, the CLIA program may be contacted directly (410-786-3531) for the address and phone number of the appropriate state agency.[5]

After the application has been submitted to the CMS state agency, the facility will receive a fee coupon assessing a fee based on the information provided in the application. The payment should be sent according to the instructions provided and can usually be paid online. Once CMS has received the fee, they will mail the CLIA Certificate of Waiver to the facility. The CLIA Certificate of Waiver contains a ten-character alpha-numeric code to be used when communicating with the state agency and CMS regarding the licensed facility. After the CLIA Certificate of Waiver has been received by the facility and all state-law requirements have been met, it is vital to notify the state board of pharmacy, as well as any other required state regulatory boards, before testing begins. Once the facility has received certification to perform tests for the purposes listed above, the facility will be considered a laboratory under state law.[5] State agencies must be notified within 30 days if there are any changes made at the facility, including, but not limited to, ownership, name, address, phone number, laboratory director, or the initiation of more complex testing.

Regulatory and Safety Considerations

CLIA requires that all waived tests be simple and have a low risk for false results, but these requirements do not mean that the tests themselves and the testing process are completely error-proof. Therefore, it is required by CLIA that the HCP complete the waived test(s) by explicitly following the manufacturer's instructions found in the package insert for each test.[5] Failure to precisely follow all manufacturer instructions found in the package insert leads to inaccurate test results, which could lead to misdiagnosis or delay in treatment. In addition to manufacturer instructions, some tests include quick-reference guides. While these guides are generally helpful, they should never be substituted for the actual step-by-step instructions provided in the package insert. Adhering to all instructions is critical for proper patient care.[5] It is also important to note that CMS conducts inspections to verify that laboratories are compliant with regulations. These inspections are conducted on a biennial basis or if CMS receives complaints alleging non-compliance.[7]

CLIA-waived laboratory testing requires the HCP to collect a sample, such as blood, in a minimally invasive manner. All CLIA-waived laboratories must comply with the Occupational Safety and Health (OSH) Act of 1970 to ensure safe and healthful working conditions for those collecting samples.[8] The bloodborne pathogens standard (29 CFR 1910.1030) of the Occupational Safety and Health Administration (OSHA), as amended pursuant to the Needlestick Safety and Prevention Act of 2000, details health-related safeguards protecting workers against the health risks caused by bloodborne pathogens.[9] A quick-reference guide to these safeguards is available for HCP.[10] The standards address items such as hazardous and non-hazardous chemical exposure control plans (example available from OSHA at www.osha.gov/sites/default/files/publications/osha3186.pdf), universal precautions, engineering and work practice controls, personal protective equipment, housekeeping, laboratories, hepatitis B vaccination, post-exposure follow-up, communication and training, records for occupational injuries and other recordkeeping (Table 2–2).[9] The hepatitis B vaccine must be offered within 10 days of employment; an employee who declines the vaccine may accept later. In addition, the standards place requirements for yearly training on organizations whose employees can be reasonably anticipated to come in contact with blood or other potentially infectious materials (OPIM), such as bodily substances including, but not limited to, blood, mucous, saliva, and urine.[10] The facility must follow all safeguards outlined in the standard to comply with federal regulations to maintain the CLIA Certificate of Waiver.[10]

Step 4: Environment

The physical environment of the laboratory should have sufficient space to ensure patient privacy and a clean work area for the testing devices with the space needed to perform testing. Other physical environment considerations include lighting, storage, temperature and humidity levels, utilities needed to conduct the test(s), and overall housekeeping of the workspace.[3,11]

Step 5: Selecting Testing Devices

Due to the nature of POCT, it is important for the health care professional who serves as the director of the laboratory to select the tests and testing devices that are most suitable for the HCP and patients. The most important considerations include the testing device characteristics, samples required to complete the test, and associated costs. Other considerations include storage requirements, temperature sensitivity, sample collection, handling of components, timing of results, range of accuracy, policies and procedures, and limitations.[3] As the facility begins adding point-of-care services, it may be beneficial to add each testing device individually to decrease overall cost and time spent on training and implementation.[3]

Table 2-2. Bloodborne pathogens standard and CLIA recordkeeping

Record	Requirements	Length
Hepatitis B vaccination	Documentation of completion of vaccine series	Length of employment plus 30 years
Hepatitis B declination	"I understand that due to my occupational exposure to blood or other potentially infectious materials I may be at risk of acquiring hepatitis B virus (HBV) infection. I have been given the opportunity to be vaccinated with hepatitis B vaccine, at no charge to myself. However, I decline hepatitis B vaccination at this time. I understand that by declining this vaccine, I continue to be at risk of acquiring hepatitis B, a serious disease. If in the future I continue to have occupational exposure to blood or other potentially infectious materials and I want to be vaccinated with hepatitis B vaccine, I can receive the vaccination series at no charge to me."	Length of employment
Sharps injury log	Date and time of the exposure Procedure or action being performed during the injury Information about the injury stated in a manner that protects the employee's confidentiality Type and brand of the device involved (if known) Department or work area in which the exposure occurred Explanation of how the exposure occurred: How deep was the injury? Did the injury occur while the employee was using a safety device? Was the protective mechanism activated?	5 years
Exposure control	Example available at CDC: https://www.cdc.gov/sharpssafety/pdf/appendixa-7.pdf	3 years
Training records	Date and completion of training	3 years
Test procedures	Manufacturer procedures	2 years
Patient testing	Test requisition and authorizations	2 years
Quality control	Initials of person performing control Date Test name, lot number, expiration date Each control level with lot # and expiration date Results of control testing	2 years
Temperature log	Temperature recorded daily	2 years

Step 6: Personnel Training

In order to ensure that POCT is conducted appropriately, all pharmacy personnel must complete the appropriate training (Table 2–3).[8] Documentation of completion of training must be maintained by the pharmacy.[8] Personnel training includes two main components: initial training and repeat competency-based training.[8] The objectives of initial training are to ensure that personnel understand the policies and procedures outlined by the pharmacy, to have proper testing procedures confirmed by a trainer, to perform all steps associated with POCT, and to document necessary components.[8] The objective of repeat competency-based training is to ensure that testing continues to be completed in an accurate, safe and effective manner for all patients.[8] In addition, having other trained personnel may increase the number of patients who can receive the clinical services offered.[12,13] Depending on state-specific laws, the personnel allowed to complete testing may vary depending upon licensure (pharmacist versus pharmacy technician) and other designated credentials.

Pharmacist and Supporting Staff Training

The specific training and frequency of completion required to ensure competency may vary depending upon state-specific laws. See Table 2–3 for information regarding general training for testing personnel.

Documentation of Training

Each pharmacy must establish a procedure for documentation surrounding orientation, personnel training, and competency/performance evaluations. This procedure must be in compliance with state laws and will likely need to include descriptions of how documentation is completed, where records are kept, and how long records must be maintained.

Step 7: Initiation of Testing

Policies and procedures for testing must be clearly outlined, including standard operating procedures for testing. Each part of the selected tests must be performed in accordance with the manufacturer's package insert, and each part should be performed in the same way by every individual testing patients. The manufacturer's instructions and/or package insert must be readily accessible within the testing area by those completing the selected POCT.[3,8] Pharmacies may decide how best to organize this information; for example, the facility could maintain a binder containing the manufacturers' instructions for each test. In addition, each pharmacy completing testing should have a procedure manual outlining the manufacturer's instructions and specific instructions for that pharmacy.[8] The CDC recommends that certain content is included within the pharmacy's procedure manual, including, but not limited to, preparing for and performing the POCT, training new personnel, disposal of testing materials, and maintaining POCT devices/equipment.[8] For a full list of content to consider for inclusion in procedure manuals, refer to the CDC's "To Test or Not to Test? Considerations for Waived Testing."[8] For additional information, refer to Chapter 3 for testing procedures and to Chapter 4 for implementation considerations.

Table 2-3. Types of training

Type of training	Additional information
OSHA's Bloodborne Pathogens	OSHA outlines standards for this training and the specific content that must be covered to meet legal requirements. Pharmacies may choose to develop their own training procedures or utilize existing training procedures from other organizations.
OSHA's Hazard Communication	
Point-of-care device testing technique	General technique training may include[8]: • Reading the test instructions • Observing POCT procedures performed by the trainer • Identification and organization of materials needed to complete the test • Performing quality control and testing • Interpreting results • Cleaning work area • Trainer evaluation of test results with feedback • Documentation as necessary Some POCTs have specific information from the manufacturer regarding testing techniques that may need to change for each device.
Point-of-care device maintenance	Pharmacy policies and procedures must outline the importance of maintenance for all POCT devices and the personnel responsible for completing maintenance. Some POCTs have specific information from the manufacturer on procedures and maintenance.
Point-of-care device troubleshooting	Pharmacy policies and procedures must outline steps to be followed if the POCT device is not working properly. Some POCTs have specific information from the manufacturer regarding troubleshooting and contact information for technical support.
Results interpretation	Each POCT may have distinct procedures for reading and interpreting results. Personnel must be familiar with the criteria for positive/negative results and invalid tests, as well as the subsequent steps to be followed for each type of result.
Billing procedures	Pharmacies may select three potential billing models: self-pay, insurance reimbursement or a combination of both. Depending upon the selected billing model, personnel may need to be trained on requirements outlined by different insurance companies (commercial plans, Medicaid, and Medicare) to ensure that reimbursement is collected by the pharmacy.

Step 8: Quality Assessment

Similar to required Continuous Quality Improvement (CQI) meetings within the community pharmacy setting, quality assessment must be performed for all POCT. Quality assessment is required to ensure the pharmacy and pharmacy personnel continue to provide quality services. The two main kinds of quality assessment are internal and external.[8] Internal assessment is performed by the pharmacy and pharmacy personnel to evaluate current procedures and practices.[8] External assessment is completed by an external organization to evaluate current procedures and practices.[8]

Quality control procedures must be performed on a regular basis and documented by pharmacy personnel. The quality control frequency for POCT may vary depending on the manufacturer's instructions. The internal assessment process should include "performing, documenting and reviewing quality control procedures and results."[8] Once this information is reviewed, the pharmacy must determine steps to improve the safety, efficacy, and efficiency of current processes.[8] External assessments are not required, but they are recommended by OSHA. For example, in proficiency testing, two samples are collected, and the pharmacy completes the test and reports the results to a proficiency testing program.[8] The proficiency testing program then completes their own test and determines if the results match.[8]

Documentation of Quality Assessments

As with all pharmacy services, documentation is vital to assess results and determine what steps should be taken if the results of the quality assessment are not within an acceptable range. Quality assessment documentation must include:[11]

- Quality control dates and results
- Equipment maintenance and evaluation based on manufacturer's instructions
- If the POCT device requires calibration, a record of completion and dates
- Patient results and procedure if results require further referral to additional health care professionals
- Pharmacy personnel training completion and dates

Conclusion

As the scope of community-based pharmacy practice continues to evolve from a dispensing based model to that of a clinically focused appointment-based profession, it is vital for pharmacies to consider implementing POCT.[14] A required component of this change is the performance of CLIA-waived tests requiring a CLIA Certificate of Waiver. While there is an application process and training program the HCP must complete, the benefits for both the pharmacy and the patients they serve far exceed the effort needed to set up the pharmacy-based CLIA-waived laboratory. Federal laws exist to allow pharmacists as HCPs to conduct CLIA-waived testing, but limitations exist due to unclear state-specific laws and regulations. A growing body of evidence demonstrates the importance of developing pharmacy-based CLIA-waived laboratories to expand clinical services to improve patient outcomes, access to care and public health efforts.[15] These services will provide communities with the care needed to address their overall health and wellness.

References

1. Centers for Medicare and Medicaid Services: Good Laboratory Practices. Available at: https://www.cms.gov/regulations-and-guidance/legislation/clia/downloads/wgoodlab.pdf. Accessed February 10, 2024

2. Garrels M, Oatis C. Laboratory Testing for Ambulatory Settings - E-Book: A Guide for Health Care Professionals. 2nd ed. Elsevier/Saunders; 2011. Accessed February 10, 2024.

3. Centers for Disease Control and Prevention. Clinical Laboratory Improvement Amendments (CLIA). Atlanta, GA: CDC. Available at: https://www.cdc.gov/clia/index.html. Accessed February 10, 2024.

4. U.S. Food and Drug Administration, Center for Devices and Radiological Health. Clinical Laboratory Improvement Amendments (CLIA). Silver Spring, MD: FDA. Available at: https://www.fda.gov/medical-devices/ivd-regulatory-assistance/clinical-laboratory-improvement-amendments-clia. Accessed February 10, 2024.

5. Centers for Medicare and Medicaid Services. Clinical Laboratory Improvement Amendments (CLIA) How to Obtain a CLIA Certificate of Waiver. Baltimore, MD: CMS. Available at: https://www.cms.gov/regulations-and-guidance/legislation/clia/downloads/howobtaincertificateofwaiver.pdf. Accessed February 10, 2024.

6. Centers for Disease Control and Prevention. Good Laboratory Practices for Waived Testing Sites. Atlanta, GA: CDC. Available at: https://www.cdc.gov/mmwr/pdf/rr/rr5413.pdf. Accessed February 10, 2024.

7. American Association of Family Physicians. CLIA Inspections. Leawood, KS: AAFP. Available at: https://www.aafp.org/family-physician/practice-and-career/managing-your-practice/clia/inspections.html. Accessed February 10, 2024.

8. Occupational Safety and Health Administration. About Occupational Safety and Health Standards. Washington, DC: OSHA. Available at: https://www.osha.gov/aboutosha. Accessed February 10, 2024.

9. Occupational Safety and Health Administration. Occupational Safety and Health Standards: 1910.1030—Bloodborne pathogens. Washington, DC: OSHA. Available at: https://www.osha.gov/laws-regs/regulations/standardnumber/1910/1910.1030. Accessed February 10, 2024.

10. Occupational Safety and Health Administration. Bloodborne Pathogens and Needlestick Prevention—Quick Reference Guide. Washington, DC: OSHA. Available at: https://www.osha.gov/bloodborne-pathogens/quick-reference. Accessed February 10, 2024.

11. Centers for Disease Control and Prevention. To Test or Not to Test? Considerations for waived testing. Atlanta, GA: CDC. Available at: https://www.cdc.gov/labquality/docs/waived-tests/15_255581-test-or-not-test-booklet.pdf. Accessed February 10, 2024.

12. Pope S, Hill H, Cardosi L, et al. Enhancing point-of-care testing through standardized training and redeployment of pharmacy technicians in the community setting. *Explor Res Clin Soc Pharm*. 2021;2:100034. doi:10.1016/j.rcsop.2021.100034

13. Hill H, Cardosi L, Henson L, et al. Evaluating advanced pharmacy technician roles in the provision of point-of-care testing. *J Am Pharm Assoc* (2003). 2020;60(4):e64–e69. doi:10.1016/j.japh.2020.02.024

14. Doucette J, Lavino J. Ability of community pharmacists to independently perform CLIA-waived testing—A multi-state legal review. Explor Res in Clin Soc Pharm. 2021;2:100024. doi:10.1016/j.rcsop.2021.100024

15. Cillessen LM, Lyons-Burney H, Gubbins PO. Pharmacist use of point-of-care testing to improve access to care. Remington. 2021:817–828. doi:10.1016/B978-0-12-820007-0.00046-5

16. U.S. Food and Drug Administration. Clinical Laboratory Improvement Amendments (CLIA). Silver Spring, MD: FDA. Available at: https://www.fda.gov/medical-devices/ivd-regulatory-assistance/clinical-laboratory-improvement-amendments-clia. Accessed February 10, 2024.

Point-of-Care Testing Protocol Development and Requirements

Bradley Van Riper, PharmD

Key Points

- A pharmacist's ability to prescribe will vary by state and will be dictated by the type of prescriptive authority granted by statute or board rule.
- The two categories of pharmacist prescribing are dependent or independent, and prescriptions may be made through collaborative practice or protocols.
- Protocols have four main parts: patient identification, documentation and communication expectations, quality assurance, and the patient care algorithm.
- Pharmacists have specific documentation requirements and established communication methods in the protocol; adhering to each of these requirements is critical to establishing trust.
- Tracking outcomes will help to determine the success of current program offerings, allow for better marketing, and identify future areas of growth.

Introduction

Pharmacists conducting point-of-care testing (POCT) can initiate, "prescribe," or manage therapy for patients pursuant to a prescription, a government protocol, a collaborative practice agreement (CPA), or standard-of-care legislative provisions. A pharmacist may conduct the POCT, notify a prescribing provider of the results, and receive a prescription order for treatment or a change in therapy. Government protocols can provide the authority for pharmacists to prescribe treatment pursuant to a POCT. Pharmacists must meet the specific criteria and follow the protocol's requirements. In addition, if not using a government protocol, pharmacists will need a CPA that creates a formal relationship between a pharmacist and prescriber and describes the scope of practice allowed by the pharmacist under the agreement. A CPA contains the scope of agreement and legal and administrative components, and it may or may not include a specific algorithm for the care of the patient.[1]

Pharmacist Prescriptive Authority

The ability of pharmacists to prescribe is typically either dependent or independent, as described in Box 3–1.[1]

Independent Category-Specific Authority

Independent category-specific prescribing authority can be thought of as an expanded scope of practice applied to specific conditions and/or medications. Examples of this type of authority include government protocols (i.e., naloxone or immunizations; Box 3-1) and federally mandated exceptions such as those enacted for COVID-19 by emergency order. Outside of the very recent innovation of standard-of-care pharmacist prescribing, this type of authority is the least restrictive.

> **Box 3–1. Requirements for government protocol***
>
> - Published by a government body pursuant to the directions of passed legislation
> - If you are a licensed pharmacist and you meet all enumerated criteria, you may follow the protocol as written
> - Most often used for preventive care or to treat self-limiting conditions
>
> Examples: state immunization or naloxone nasal spray protocol
>
> *Notably, in this context, "protocol" implies a broad application suitable for any pharmacist that meets the basic criteria mentioned. As described below, the concept of a "protocol" is in the context of a CPA. In the latter, the rules are more restrictive and usually accompanied by a treatment algorithm.

Independent Standard-of-Care Pharmacist Prescribing

As of 2024, only Colorado, Idaho, and Montana have implemented standard-of-care pharmacist prescribing. In this system, pharmacists are limited only by the requirement to adhere to what would be considered the standard of care for treatment of a particular condition by other pharmacists in a similar clinical situation (Table 3–1). While intentionally vague to broaden access to care, this approach may increase liability concerns for pharmacists.

Table 3–1. Non-diagnostic and diagnostic standard-of-care prescribing

Non-diagnostic	• A previous diagnosis is required • May prescribe preventive or add-on therapy for conditions that were previously diagnosed

Diagnostic	• Pharmacist may be first to provide diagnosis of the condition to be treated
	    • **Targeted:** Pharmacists are given a list of conditions/circumstances that allow them to diagnose and prescribe
	    • **Open-ended:** The ability to prescribe is included in the pharmacy practice act

Dependent Collaborative Practice Agreement

CPAs can expand a pharmacist's scope of practice by allowing them to enter into an agreement with a prescriber to work within a mutually agreed upon protocol. CPAs may range in restrictiveness as described in Table 3–2.[1,6]

Table 3–2. Characteristics of patient- and population-specific CPAs

Patient-specific CPA	• Most restrictive • Often used for chronic disease state management • Example: "Pharmacist may treat hyperlipidemia according to the enclosed treatment algorithm for any of Dr. Johnson's patients whom he specifically refers using the form 'Dr. Johnson Hyperlipidemia Management Pharmacist Referral'" • Only patients of the prescriber with whom one has an agreement are eligible for treatment in this instance
Population-specific CPA	• Used to provide care to a patient population regardless of the identity of the patient's HCP • Works well in acute care situations • Example: "Pharmacist may test and treat any patient >18 years old that presents with signs/symptoms of influenza"
Unrestricted category-specific authority	• Least restrictive • Pharmacist may prescribe medication(s) within their regularly defined scope of practice • Example: The state publishes a list of medications that pharmacists may prescribe with no further direction/limitations presented

A protocol is used in medicine to describe a systematic plan for providing care for patients. The protocol within a CPA will include all areas necessary to provide a clear explanation of the agreement being entered into (see Figure 3–1). However, the term protocol is sometimes used interchangeably with a particular portion of the protocol called the treatment algorithm or patient care plan. Protocol development will ultimately "make or break" point-of-care services, regardless of practice setting. If your protocol is too restrictive, there is a real risk of limiting your eligible patient population to the point of financial unviability. Conversely, if your protocol provides no limits, there will need to be a great deal of trust in the clinical capabilities of all those operating under its instruction. The protocol's wording is of equal importance to the personnel involved in its development. Choosing a collaborating HCP personally known to the pharmacist may remove layers of accountability that could prove necessary for the proper administration and monitoring of the service provided. However, choosing a collaborating provider unknown to the pharmacist will be more difficult and may limit their ability to provide meaningful services to your patients.

Finding a Collaborating Provider

There are two main paths to finding a provider with whom to enter into an agreement, as described in Table 3–3. The first path involves organic relationships that are made in the community and using personal interactions to get buy-in from a local provider, which can seem like a daunting and time-consuming process. Alternatively, many companies (Cardinal Health, Scripted, etc.) offer pre-arranged contracts with providers that they have identified, which can be easy to set up and can get services up and running quickly. There are pros and cons to either approach. Verify state-specific requirements regarding an acceptable prescriber partner. Some states do not allow advanced practice providers, like nurse practitioners or physicians' assistants, to enter into a CPA.

Table 3–3. Paths to provider collaborations

Organically developed relationship	**Pros:** • Both parties are familiar with each other, which can offer improved trust from the beginning • The initial PCP can be a champion of your services to others in the community when positive outcomes are demonstrated • Any issues that arise can be resolved quickly • Mutual referrals can help the business of both parties
	Cons: • A greater amount of time is needed to set up the agreement • PCP may demand more from the agreement in terms of access to outcomes data than the HCP is willing to provide • "Reinventing the wheel" with each new provider engaged with or service offered
Wholesaler agreement	**Pros:** • Easy to set up and services can begin to be offered quickly • PCP is not likely to want a lot of communication back and forth as they may be entering into multiple agreements over a large area • "Cut and paste" method may be good for expanding to multiple locations or adding services over time
	Cons: • "Cookie cutter" agreements that may not meet the specific needs of your business • Conflicts may be more difficult to resolve • Little or no ability to communicate directly with the PCP • Making changes as experience dictates over time may not be possible • Relatively high cost

Key: HCP, health care provider; PCP, primary care physician.

One potentially beneficial strategy to be considered is not limiting oneself to a single provider for a given service offering. For example, for influenza, a potential scenario is as follows:

- Provider #1 is a family practice physician, and the agreement covers patients aged 12 and up
- Provider #2 is a pediatrician, whose agreement covers patients from 1 to 11 years old
- Provider #3 is an obstetrician, whose agreement covers pregnant and nursing patients

By utilizing such a system, the patient base can be expanded, and help can be offered to additional areas of the community.

If a pharmacist is operating under a government protocol, a collaborating HCP is not necessary. The government protocol will include all necessary components to guide the pharmacist providing care for patients.

Figure 3–1. Necessary components of a point-of-care protocol[3]

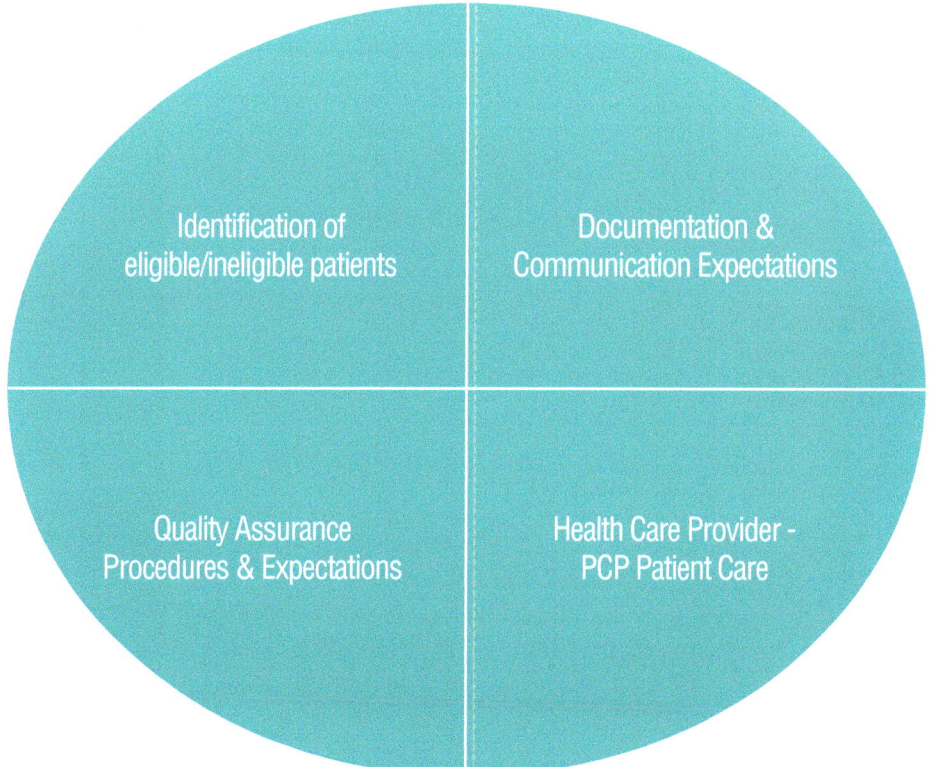

Identification of Eligible and Ineligible Patients[3]

This first step in identifying eligible and ineligible patients is defining the target patient population. Only patients deemed eligible by the protocol should be tested and treated. Services provided to patients outside of those allowed by protocol may not be covered by liability insurance. Additionally, beyond just the wording of the protocol, pharmacists should consider their own expertise and degree of comfort with each service before expanding their scope of practice. Regardless of the practice site, this program will become part of the practice's business model. With that in mind, if eligibility is limited to an excessive degree, the return on investment (ROI) will be limited as well. Conversely, if there are too few exclusions to treatment, workflows and individual workloads may become stressed and potential liability will be increased.

Identifying patients that are eligible or ineligible can be accomplished using a construct with which health care professionals are familiar. Inclusion and exclusion criteria, like those used for research studies, are helpful in this regard. Some criteria to consider (though not intended to be exhaustive) are summarized in Figure 3–2.

Figure 3–2. Criteria to consider in determining patient eligibility

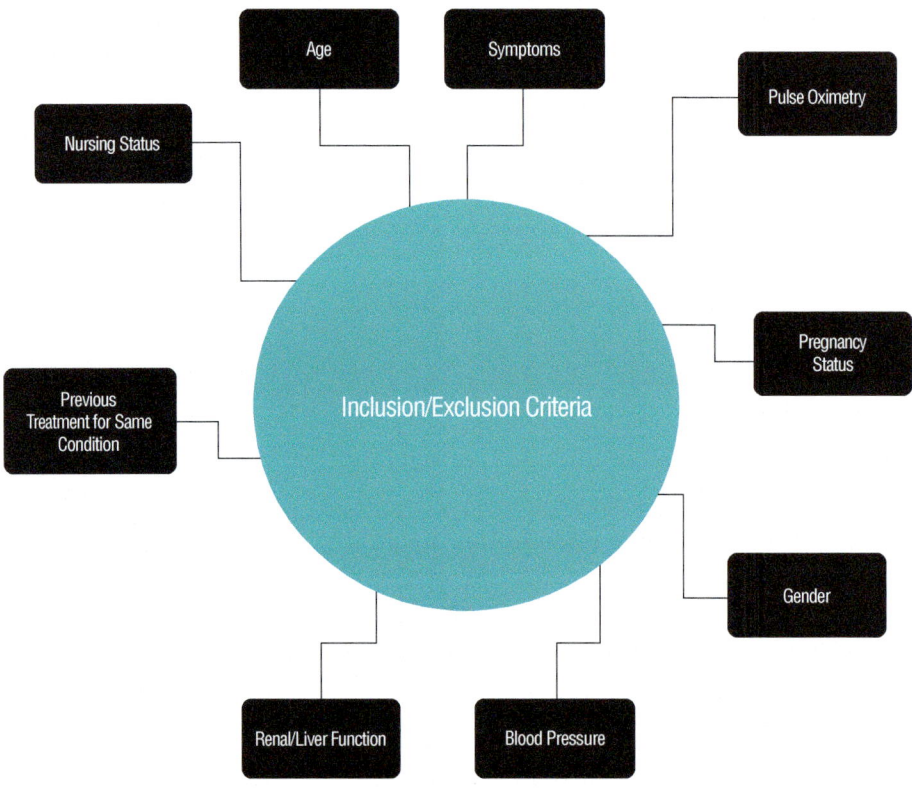

An example protocol section of this type is included in Box 3-2 below.

Box 3-2. Treatment Criteria for Group A Strep[4]

A patient presenting to a pharmacist at Elsie's Family Pharmacy for evaluation and potential treatment for group A strep ("Strep Throat") shall first be screened using the following measures:

Inclusion Criteria

- >3 years old
- Symptoms consistent with strep throat
- Ability to safely tolerate an oropharyngeal swab
- Consent given for an examination of the oral cavity

Exclusion Criteria

- <3 years old
- Signs or symptoms of Scarlet or Rheumatic Fever
- Rash, "strawberry tongue," joint pain
- Unwillingness or intolerability of mouth exam and oropharyngeal swab
- Allergic to or intolerability of all first, second, and third line therapies as defined in the patient care algorithm
- Treatment for the same condition within the last 30 days

Should a patient meet all inclusion criteria and none of the exclusion criteria, the pharmacist may proceed with the test-and-treat program as further defined in this protocol.

Documentation and Communication Expectations[2]

As pharmacists begin to assert themselves into treatment realms traditionally reserved for PCPs, building trust with the collaborating PCP is essential to establishing mutual respect. The most basic form of trust that can be established is simply following through on what was agreed upon. Setting clear expectations that meet the needs of the PCP while not being overly burdensome to the pharmacist will ensure satisfaction for both. Consult state requirements before entering into a collaboration, as each will be unique. If following a statewide protocol, documentation and communication expectations will be included in the protocol. When establishing the particulars for your agreement, consider the following.

Documentation

- Where must documentation be stored?
- Will the documentation be hard copies or electronic?
- For how long must the records be kept?
- Who must/should have a copy of the records?
- Will the PCP receive a copy of every encounter, a summary of encounters, or encounter information only upon request?

Communication

- Primarily, determine what communication is required versus wanted.
- If the originally agreed upon expiration date of the agreement is approaching, a meeting must occur to confirm continuation of the partnership or its termination.
- Would the PCP like to meet occasionally to discuss the success of the agreement or any barriers to success that have occurred?
- If so, will the meeting be in person, on the phone, through an email exchange, or virtually?
- If successful, should other PCPs be included in the call so the original PCP can act as a champion for the program and your clinical services?
- Should communication occur weekly, monthly, or yearly? Should communication be more frequent at first then gradually decline in frequency as trust is built?
- The form of communication should be specified as well: telephone, fax, email, or documented in the electronic health record.
- If any patient-specific information is included in your communications, then HIPAA-compliant technology must be employed.

An example protocol section of this type is included in Box 3–3 below.

Box 3–3. Documentation and Communication

The HCP performing test-and-treat services at Elsie's Family Pharmacy will keep a written record of each encounter. For this agreement's purposes, that record shall be stored electronically on the pharmacy management system. All documentation must be kept for at least 5 years from the last service date. If the patient was not previously associated with the pharmacy, then a Health Insurance Portability and Accountability Act (HIPAA) form must be signed and kept on record. At a minimum, the documentation must include:
- Date of birth
- Sex
- Health conditions
- Blood pressure/pulse
- List of current medications
- Description of presenting symptoms
- Results of any test(s) performed
- Assessment of the patient's condition
- Plan for treatment and follow-up

To make sure the agreement continues to meet the needs of both parties, a virtual or in-person meeting will occur once a year. Between meetings, communication will be conducted as needed for either party. Minimally, the agenda for each meeting shall include:
- Open discussion concerning how well each party feels the agreement is working
- Any changes to the agreement that should be made
- Decision to continue or terminate the agreement
- Share feedback received from patients on either side

Quality Assurance Procedures and Expectations

Quality assurance can be thought about as two distinct categories: procedural quality and quality of care.

Procedural Quality

Each testing device has specific instructions for performing quality assurance measures. Failure to follow these procedures may result in inaccurate test results/improper patient care. It is important that each individual responsible for using the equipment is familiar with maintaining quality standards for each procedure. The "quick start guide" included with most testing equipment should never be used as the basis for quality assurance policies; the instructions should be read completely to ensure that all crucial details are considered. Once the quality procedures are understood, documentation that the facility is following through on these procedures should be stored in a central location.

Although equipment quality assurance procedures are discussed in detail in Chapter 2, a brief synopsis is included here. Typically, equipment quality control measures will fall into one of two categories: external or internal.

External

External quality assurance measures are typified by the use of a test kit to perform a test against a predetermined standard. Depending on the equipment, this procedure could be a single test, a "high" and a "low" test, a "positive" and a "negative" test, or multiple tests as defined by the manufacturer. Regardless of the specific procedure for an individual piece of equipment, the results of these quality assurance tests must be documented, maintained, and kept available for inspection.

Internal

Some test devices are equipped with a software program and/or a reusable "test kit" that allows for quality control measures to be conducted with minimal expense and time investment. When performing quality control procedures for such devices, it is important that the manufacturer's instructions are followed and documentation is kept in an easily accessible place.

Although a full discussion of costs is outside of this chapter's scope, the cost of performing quality control procedures should be incorporated into the business plan as a part of the overall cost of doing business.

Quality of Care

Procedures to measure the quality of the care provided by a facility may be included in the protocol or in a separate reference document. Some states require outcomes data to be collected, but this is not always the case. Even when it is not required by law, analysis of outcomes data can serve as a useful tool to measure ROI and the effectiveness of the care being provided. Quality of care can also be broken down into two categories: outcomes and patient satisfaction.

Outcomes

As the cost, procedures, required physical space overhaul, and timeline of changes of new testing and treatment procedures are determined, a decision should be made as to whether outcomes data will be kept, either now or in the future. Outcomes data may be beneficial in the following ways:

- Evaluating the success of your business model
- Determining impact on your community
- Evaluating equipment selection
- Identifying potential tests for the future

Types of data that could be considered for collection include:

- Number of each test completed
- Time to perform each test
- Revenue generated
- Percent of test kits used before expiration
- Number of positive/negative tests
- Number of positive/negative tests vs stated specificity/sensitivity
- If possible, percent of your positive patients that eventually utilized the emergency department versus state or local averages

Patient Satisfaction

While most HCPs want to know if the services they provide are resulting in benefit to patients, it may be beneficial in some circumstances to share that data with the PCP. Presumably, the PCP sees potential benefit to their patients as a result of your services, and it may be beneficial to demonstrate that they were correct. Aside from reassuring the PCP, other reasons why these data might be useful include:

- Providing evidence to potential third-party payors
- Self-promotion/advertising materials
- Promotion to local employers/media
- Proof of concept when considering additional services to offer

Patient satisfaction data could be obtained using several different methods. Regardless of the chosen data collection method, it is important that the information can be turned around quickly to keep marketing strategies and advertising campaigns current. Some of the ways in which data can be collected include:

- Paper-based satisfaction surveys
- Digital surveys sent to patients
- Point-of-sale questions to gauge patient experiences
- Hiring a third-party vendor to monitor social media and/or create tools to track how referrals are being received
- Referral question on patient check-in forms
- Track and attempt to improve your star-rating on Google.com or other "review" websites

An example protocol section of this type is included Box 3–4 below.

> **Box 3–4**
>
> Elsie's Family Pharmacy shall maintain quality control records for each testing device according to complete manufacturer instructions and applicable state statutes/rules. These records shall include control tests, inspection reports, cleaning logs, maintenance records, and any other device-specific documentation. The PCP shall have access to these records upon written request. Notice shall be provided at least 48 hours in advance to allow for the collection and organization of the records for inspection.
>
> Elsie's Family Pharmacy shall collect outcomes and patient satisfaction data at their own discretion. If data is collected, however, a summary of that data shall be provided to the PCP quarterly for the first year and annually thereafter. This summary shall be sent via secure fax to the PCP's office.

Patient Care Algorithm[3-5]

This portion of the protocol will be the most specific and comprehensive. Combined with the inclusion and exclusion criteria, the algorithm will determine exactly which treatments the HCP may prescribe and other actions that they may/must take. Some portions of the protocol may be dictated by state statute or board rule, while others will be determined by health care provider-PCP agreement.

As you develop your protocol, keep in mind that maintaining financial feasibility is important. The less restrictive your exclusion criteria are, and the more options are listed as approved treatments, the larger the potential patient base will be. Maximizing the patient base will provide financial benefits and enhance a pharmacist's ability to highlight their services firsthand. A straightforward way to keep this in the forefront of your thought process is to remember: "turning them away may just turn them off."

Each protocol will differ in the specific components of its algorithm due to the many variables present. Some variables that will influence the ultimate design of the algorithm include:

- State statutes
- Board rules
- PCP comfort level
- HCP comfort level
- Treatment guidelines
- Liability concerns
- Payment potential

A simplified algorithm for group A strep is presented in Figure 3–3. Keep in mind that specific algorithms may be more or less comprehensive based on the criteria previously identified.

Figure 3–3. Sample patient care algorithm

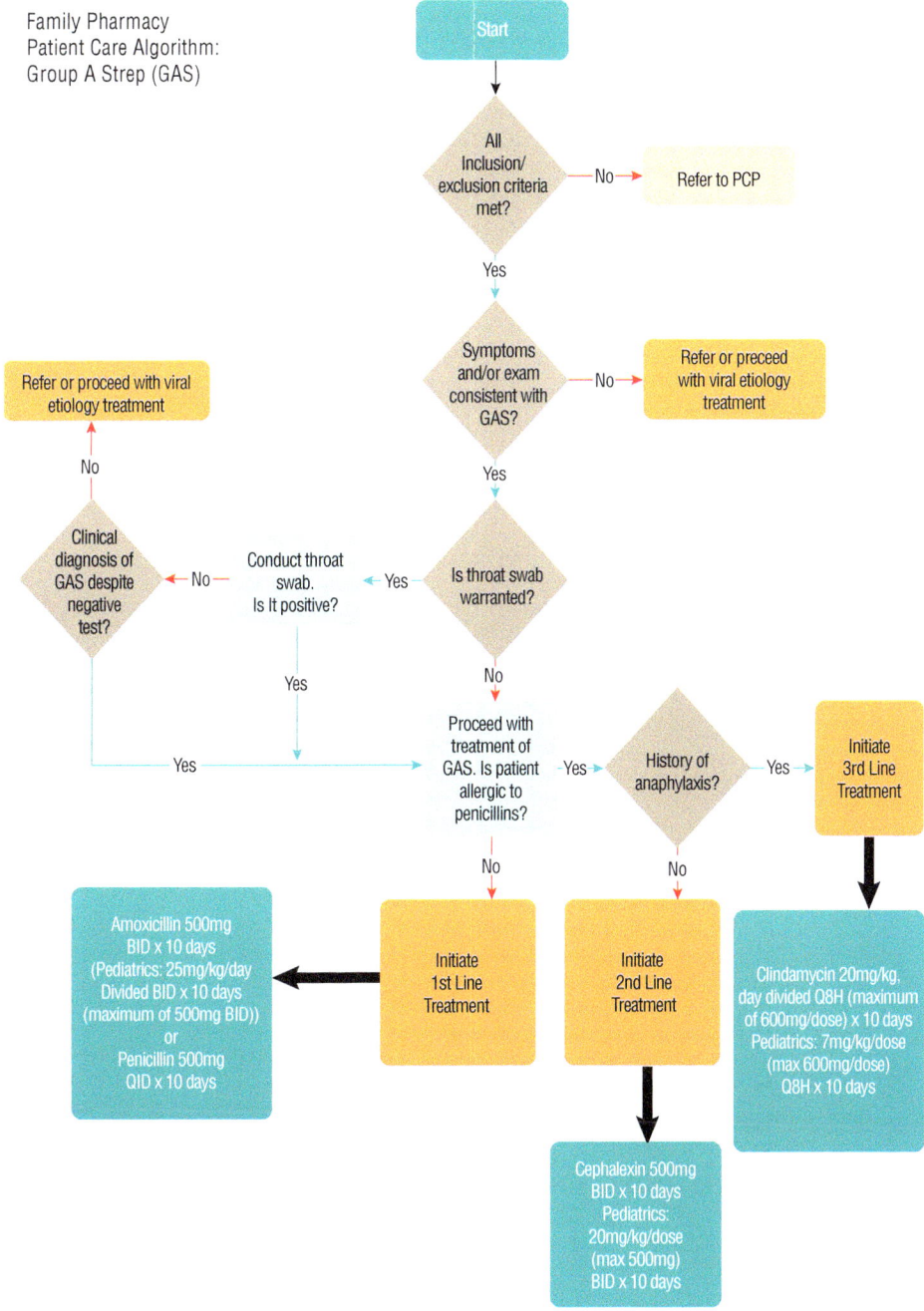

Conclusion

Determining the potential patient base, establishing sound quality measurements, setting clear expectations, and choosing an appropriate practitioner with whom to partner with will determine the success of any newly established POCT program. The document, or protocol, that codifies the specifics agreed upon may be labor intensive to create but will provide clear direction and practices to maximize the chances of achieving that success. As trust is built with one partner, new partners and opportunities to expand the scope of practice will follow. Protocol development is a learned skill and will improve with repeated attempts and regular assessment of current protocols in place.

References

1. Centers for Disease Control and Prevention. Advancing Team-Based Care Through Collaborative Practice Agreements: A Resource and Implementation Guide for Adding Pharmacists to the Care Team. Atlanta, GA: CDC. Department of Health and Human Services; 2017.

2. Adams AJ, Weaver KK, Adams JA. Revisiting the continuum of pharmacist prescriptive authority. *J Am Pharm Assoc*. 2023;Sep-Oct;63(5):1508–1514. doi:10.1016/j.japh.2023.06.025.

3. Adams AJ, Weaver KK. The Continuum of Pharmacist Prescriptive Authority. *Ann Pharmacother*. 2016; 50(9):778–784. doi:10.1177/1060028016653608

4. Beardsley R. Communication Skills in Pharmacy Practice. New York, NY: Lippincott Williams & Wilkins; 2012.

5. Centers for Disease Control and Prevention. Group A Streptococcal (GAS) Disease: For Clinicians. Atlanta, GA: CDC. 2016.

6. Murphy PB, Bistas KG, Le JK. Clindamycin. [Updated 2023 May 23]. In: StatPearls [Internet]. Treasure Island (FL): StatPearls Publishing; 2024 Jan. Available at: https://www.ncbi.nlm.nih.gov/books/NBK519574/. Accessed August 9, 2024.

7. Sachdev G, Kliethermes MA, Vernon V, et al. Current status of prescriptive authority by pharmacists in the United States. *J Am Coll Clin Pharm*. 2020;3(4): 807–817.

CHAPTER 4

Building a Sustainable Business Model for Point-of-Care Testing Services

Sharon Gatewood, PharmD, BCACP, FAPhA and
Deanna Tran, PharmD, BCACP, FAPhA

Key Points

- Pharmacists in point-of-care testing (POCT) services can serve in the role of advocacy and education, facilitation, and testing.
- The core components of a business plan include a description of the business and service, marketing plan, financial plan, management team, and operations.
- Tools used to receive payment for POCT services include direct patient payment, contract-based payment, incident-to-physician services, and procedural codes.

Introduction

Innovative POCT services are becoming more common in the community pharmacy setting, as there is increased demand for access to primary care services that are convenient and can be completed quickly. The increase in regulations and statewide protocols that has occurred among states to increase the scope of a pharmacist has made POCT services more common. In order for these services to be successful, they must be developed from a sustainable business model.

Pharmacy Point-of-Care Testing Business Models

State and federal regulations must be followed, including to what extent a pharmacist, a student pharmacist, and a technician can provide POCT and treatments. The foundation of this type of service is based on the pharmacists' scope of practice, including whether the pharmacist can conduct the POCT and prescribe medication, and whether the service requires a CPA or a statewide or standing protocol, as described in Chapter 3.

There are three roles for pharmacists in POCT services: advocacy and education, facilitation, and testing.[1] There are two main pathways for POCT models. In the first pathway, the pharmacist facilitates the testing process, evaluates the patient, provides treatment if applicable, and then conducts follow-up with the provider. In the second pathway, the provider assesses the patient and then refers them to the pharmacist for testing. However, within these pathways, different models may be created. In Figure 4–1, the patient enters the testing process by walking into a pharmacy or making an appointment with the pharmacist. The patient is assessed with the screening criteria either online or in person, after which the pharmacist performs the test and interprets the results for the patient. The pharmacist sends the results to the provider and the patient makes an appointment with the provider to review results and treatment. Afterwards, the patient may follow up with the pharmacist or the provider. The model shown in Figure 4–2 is mostly the same as that shown in Figure 4–1, with the only difference being where the lab test is processed. Processing of the lab test could be done by the pharmacist, or it could be outsourced through a collaboration with an outside laboratory. These two models allow the POCT to be performed at the pharmacy, which may be more accessible to patients due to proximity and hours of operation.

In Figure 4–3, the patient care process begins with the provider assessing the patient and determining if they meet the criteria for the lab test. Then the provider will refer the patient to a pharmacy where the pharmacist will perform the test. The pharmacist will interpret the results for the patient and send the results to the provider. If there is an existing collaboration between this provider and pharmacist, then the patient may continue to meet with the pharmacist for disease management. As in Figure 4–2, this model could also lead to a collaboration with an outside laboratory to process the test and send back the results to the pharmacist or the provider. In Figures 4–1 through 4–3, pharmacists are involved in all three roles: advocacy and education, facilitation, and testing.

The fourth model allows for the possibility of developing a collaboration with outside partners to come into the pharmacy location to perform POCT services. The pharmacy would provide the space for these services to take place and access for the patients to these services. There may be a cost associated with the space that is being provided to outside partners. The pharmacist is not involved in this model of testing; the pharmacist would only be involved in the roles of advocacy, education, and facilitation for the POCT service.

Figure 4–1. Advocacy and education

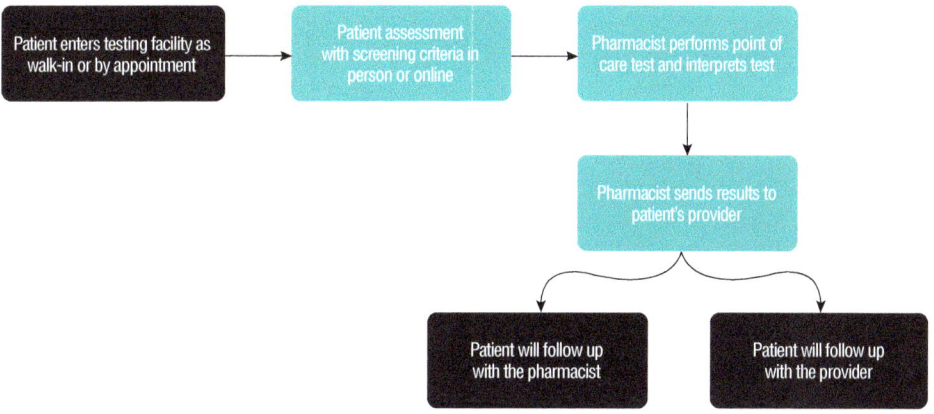

Figure 4–2. Facilitation

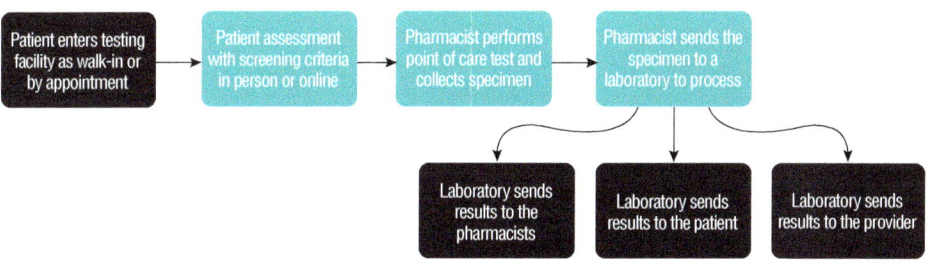

Figure 4–3. Testing

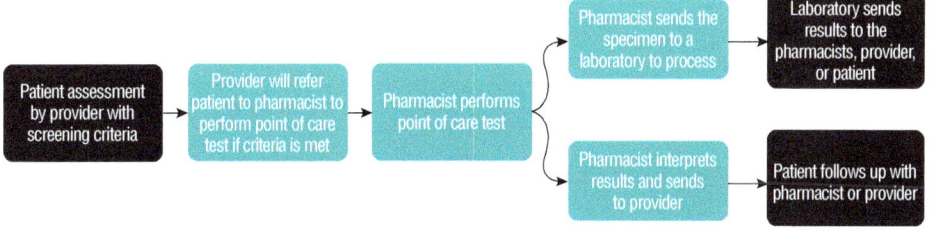

Considerations for Sustainable Business Models

A business plan may be helpful, but may be unnecessary, when creating a POCT service to create operational and financial sustainability. The core components of a business plan include a description of the business and service, marketing plan, financial plan, management team, and operations.[2] Of note, promotion of the POCT service via the marketing plan has been identified as a key facilitator of successful POCT services, as patient awareness of pharmacy-based POCT services is limited in most areas of the country.[3] Other key considerations are developing partnerships to strengthen this service, determining a range of tests that would be beneficial to the patient and providers, and designing the workflow that is necessary to implement the POCT service.[2] Two main models, a SWOT (strengths, weaknesses, opportunities, threats) analysis and the Business Model Canvas, can be used to ensure that these core components are incorporated. A SWOT analysis involves evaluating the strengths, weaknesses, opportunities, and threats regarding the business proposal. The Business Model Canvas components are the following: value proposition, customer segmenting, customer relationships, channels, key resources, key activities, core structure, and revenue streams.[4]

SWOT

A successful and sustainable business model requires assessing the surrounding pharmacy environment, which should include a thorough SWOT analysis to help the pharmacist identify the strengths, weaknesses, opportunities, and threats surrounding implementing a new POCT service.[2,5] Strengths and weaknesses are internal factors, whereas opportunities and threats are external factors. To complete a thorough SWOT, a market analysis is also needed. This analysis should include determining the demographic information of the pharmacy/clinic's current and possible future patients. Figure 4–4 shows an example of a SWOT analysis.

Figure 4–4. Example SWOT for a business conducting A1C and blood glucose testing in a community pharmacy

Strengths	Weaknesses
• Strong relationship with current patients • Patients are willing to try new services of the pharmacy • Patients have asked for this service	• No prescribing authority at the pharmacy to make changes to medications (that urgent care and emergency department/hospital could do) • CLIA-waved A1C test by a pharmacist is still a screening, not diagnosis of prediabetes or diabetes
Opportunities	Threats
• Located in a rural city that is a care desert	• An urgent care facility that could do A1C/BG testing • An emergency department and hospital in the city that could do A1C/BG testing

Business Model Canvas

The Business Model Canvas (BMC) is a strategic management tool that is used to visualize a business concept. The nine key elements of a BMC are valuable considerations in building a business plan: value proposition, customer segmenting, customer relationships, channels, key resources, key partners, key activities, cost structure, and revenue streams.[4]

The value proposition of a service communicates why a customer should utilize the pharmacy's POCT service and how it assists with customers' needs. The POCT service's value proposition should leverage the cost-effectiveness of a test, as well as its ability to deliver rapid results and provide more mobility and flexibility for patients.[6] An example value proposition statement for a grocery store chain, Safeway Pharmacy, is "the medication you need, minus the hassle." The statement is clear and effective for customers, and it highlights that it is convenient to come to the pharmacy to get tested and receive treatment medication.

Next is customer segmenting, which is the practice of finding the target audience(s) that matches the value proposition.[6] Customer segmenting also helps to gauge the service's market size to estimate how much product and supplies to order. Another related BMC component is customer relationships, in which the points of engagement between the pharmacy and its customers are outlined.[6] An example of customer relationships is services delivered at the pharmacy store, via delivery, drive through, call center service, telemedicine service, phone, and outreach events. Utilizing customer relationships and their preferences for engagement can help to narrow how the POCT service should be delivered.

A needs assessment could be conducted to help shape the value proposition and customer segment(s). This could be completed via focus groups and surveys of the pharmacy's current customers, as well as reviewing the pharmacy's electronic health record (EHR) to determine the most common disease states/infectious diseases that require more access to care. Reviewing the United States Census, working with the local health department, and surveying the community could also help to identify the unmet needs of the community (who are not current customers of the pharmacy).

Another BMC element is channels, which are defined as methods to reach and engage customers to communicate the value proposition.[6] Examples of channels include social media, word of mouth, emails, community outreach, and offline advertising such as billboards and radio. Identifying channels ultimately helps to define the service's marketing plan. Marketing of a pharmacy service often occurs at the end of the service's development. Marketing tools can be costly; the pharmacy team should balance costs with the potential impact of a marketing campaign. Word of mouth from individuals who know of the service or were provided the service is often most effective and has minimal to no financial investment. General marketing messages that are unique to POCT test-and-treat services could include:

- Convenience
- Speed at which the service is completed
- Availability after-hours (pharmacies are often open later than a traditional provider's office)
- Increase in access to care (reaching a larger pool of underserved patients that may need care)

The next consideration is determining the key resources needed to run the service, including both tangible and intangible items. Tangible items include, but are not limited to, physical space, supplies, computer/information systems to transmit patient data, and manpower/staffing needed.[4] A list of general POCT supplies are listed in Box 4–1. More supplies may be needed depending on the specific test that is being done. Make sure to review the testing procedures per the manufacturer to know what supplies are needed to perform the test.

> **Box 4–1. General list of supplies for POCT**
>
> - Absorbent pad to cover your workspace
> - Disposable gloves
> - Hand sanitizer, if applicable
> - Sharps disposal container/biohazard disposal bag
> - Alcohol swabs
> - Blood products such as cotton balls or gauze pads
> - Personal protective equipment (PPE) if applicable: face masks or coverings, particulate respirators, face shields, goggles, medical gowns

When choosing between POCT manufacturers and products, it is important to balance cost with the benefits of a particular test. There are vast differences among products, such as the type and number of tests a machine could run and whether multiple types of tests can be performed simultaneously (e.g., a test strip could run both blood sugar and a full lipid panel). The shelf life of testing supplies is crucial if relatively few tests are being conducted. The time to obtain results is important when considering workflow, staffing costs, and patient satisfaction. Products that have a quick turnaround time to a test result are often more expensive. Ultimately, product selection is tied heavily to customer segmenting and the needs assessment. To learn more about a specific product's information, refer to the product's procedure manual or reach out to the manufacturer's representatives.[5] Box 4–2 outlines core POCT product considerations.

Physical space, another tangible resource, is important for a patient-focused POCT service. Testing should be performed in a separate area where patient privacy can be maintained, tests can be conducted per the manufacturer's guidelines, any emergency safety concerns can be considered (e.g., hard surface for CPR), and proper pre- and post-test education can be provided with minimal disruptions. When providing the test in a nontraditional setting, factors such as humidity, temperature, and lighting should also be considered. Extreme humidity and temperatures may disrupt tests, while inadequate lighting may negatively impact test collection. Space should also be allocated for patient intake (e.g., filling out any screening forms, waiting to get the test, or waiting for a result).

Intangible key resources may include the required clinical knowledge and competencies to execute the service, required training to accurately utilize the POCT device, as well as required training and continuing education hours as required by federal and state law. To ensure compliance, pharmacy staff should stay up to date and in compliance with federal and state laws and regulations. For example, individuals using POCT are federally required to undergo initial and annual OSHA blood borne pathogen training.[7] In Florida, for example, pharmacists

> **Box 4–2. Considerations when choosing a particular manufacturer for POCT**
>
> - Accuracy, precision, sensitivity, specificity
> - Types of measurements that can be run in a single test that meet the needs of your customers (e.g., one test strip could check full lipid panel and blood glucose)
> - Size and portability
> - Length of time to perform a test
> - Length of time to obtain a result
> - Simplicity of operating the system
> - Required supplies to provide the test
> - Required supplies to control and calibrate
> - Shelf life of testing supplies
> - Required frequency of control tests and any supplemental tests

must complete an initial 20-hour course approved by the board to conduct test and screening services for minor non-chronic health conditions. Pharmacy owners may also want to determine what training is required for staff. Staff can stay up to date on relevant clinical knowledge, including the treatment and screening guidelines regarding the POCT being offered, through various continuing education programs.

Training on the POCT devices is also important; for example, pharmacy staff may be required to complete the PTS Diagnostics CardioChek PA device's 20-part training video and an online quiz. Lastly, required training for staff should also include reviewing any pertinent policies and procedures and relevant workflow.

As mentioned previously, it is important to establish local key partners in a POCT service. Based on state regulations, a provider may be needed for a CPA or protocol, and/or a laboratory partner may be needed to collect the sample for a POCT. Collaborations could also include student pharmacists and pharmacy residents which may provide valuable experiences for learners and potentially reduce the pharmacy staff's workload.[5] Therefore, local partners can be helpful in determining workflows, payment, and business models.

Key activities, often described as the service's workflow, describe the steps that the pharmacy needs to take in order to deliver the service's value proposition. A clear workflow ensures that the delivery of the service is efficient, effective, and safe.[8] Figures 4–1 through 4–3 describe possible workflow processes. Workflow components may include:

- Patient intake/screening
- Payment for service
- Pharmacist assessment
- Physical assessment (if applicable)
- Exclusions to treatment
- Preparation of tests
- Specimen collection
- Interpretation of results
- Patient education
- Interpretation of results
- Non-pharmacological therapies (if applicable)
- When to seek medical attention
- Documentation
- Required communication to partners, providers, etc. (if applicable)
- Required follow-up with patient (if applicable)

Considerations in the workflow may include:

- Where in the workflow are collaborators incorporated?
- Clear delineation of roles and responsibilities for pharmacy technicians, pharmacy interns (if available), and pharmacists.
- Is this service through an appointment and/or walk-in?
- Is this service incorporated into the prescription dispensing workflow or is it a separate process outside of the dispensing workflow?
- Is it available when the pharmacy is open or at certain times?
- How could service materials be organized to ensure safety and accuracy? For example, various testing materials could be color-coded, stored in separate areas in the pharmacy, and have signage.
- Good laboratory practices should be embedded into the workflow procedures.

The last two BMC components are cost structure (listing the costs incurred to deliver the service) and revenue streams (strategies to get reimbursed for the service).

Billing and payment for patient services could be billed through the medical or pharmacy insurance benefits. Medical billing uses the International Classification of Diseases (ICD) 10 codes to classify all diagnoses, symptoms, and procedures that are being billed to the insurance. Current Procedural Terminology (CPT) identifies the service being provided and is used to bill both medical and pharmacy insurances.

Payment for POCT services is a critical factor for the sustainability of the service provided by a pharmacist.[9] Recognition and payment for pharmacist patient care services has improved and advanced; the methods of billing maybe be different depending on the state, process of care, and practice setting, which may make it difficult for pharmacists to receive payment for patient care services. Payment for these services must include payment for the test, the administration of the test, and the staff time for performing the test.[10] Models used to receive payment for POCT services include direct patient payment (i.e., "cash pay"), contract-based payment, incident-to-physician services, and procedural codes. If the payer recognizes the pharmacist as the provider, the pharmacist can bill for the patient services using the pharmacist's National Provider Identifier (NPI). If the pharmacist is not recognized as a provider by the payor, then the payor can be billed by the physician or the nonphysician practitioner (NPP) and receive a portion of the payment.[11] Direct payment models are also prevalent and can be successful, with most patients willing to pay $50 or more for the service.[12]

Direct patient payment may be made out-of-pocket from the patient or through their health savings account. Contract-based payment may involve an agreement between the pharmacist and a physician or NPP, with the payment predetermined by what percentage will go to which entity. For incident-to-physician services, evaluation and management CPT codes 99211–99215, payment can be made under direct supervision or general supervision depending on the service being provided; this type of billing would be to Medicare part B or private sector medical insurance. To bill POCT services using these codes, the service provided by the pharmacist must be part of a larger service that includes history, examination, and medical decision making. The complexity of the visit would determine the level that is billed. Other procedural codes can be used, but these would be specific to the POCT test services that are being provided, such as an A1C test for a diabetes management appointment.

Quality Assessment and Evaluation

Frequent evaluation of the service is important for its long-term success. Evaluation should be more frequent with its initial implementation to determine if short-term goals are met, to address barriers to implementation, including workflow concerns, and to ensure patient and community partner satisfaction. Meanwhile, regular evaluation of a long-term service allows for improvement in efficiency and helps to ensure that long-term goals, such as clinical and financial outcomes, are met. Evaluation could also include patient and provider satisfaction, especially if there is a partnership with the provider. This data could be used to help identify needs and barriers to improve the POCT service being provided.

Conclusion

Pharmacist-provided POCT services are growing in popularity due to the need for convenient access to care for patients and developing partnerships between pharmacies and providers. Developing a strong business model for the POCT service is key to the sustainability of these services.

References

1. American Pharmacists Association. Guidelines for pharmacy-based immunization advocacy and administration. Washington, DC: APhA. Available at: https://aphanet.pharmacist.com/sites/default/files/files/Guidelines_for_Pharmacy_Based_IMZ_Advocacy_Approved_Jan_26_2019.pdf. Accessed February 11, 2204.
2. American Pharmacists Association. Writing a Business Plan for a New Pharmacy Service. The Dynamics of Pharmaceutical Care: Enriching Patients' Health. Washington, DC: APhA. Available at: https://aphanet.pharmacist.com/sites/default/files/files/mtm_writing_business_plan.pdf. Accessed February 11, 2024.
3. Hohmeier KC, McKeirnan K, Akers J, et al. Implementing community pharmacy-based influenza point-of-care test-and-treat under collaborative practice agreement. *Implementation Science Communications*. 2022 Dec;3(1):1–7.
4. Pontinha VM, Wagner TD, Holdford DA. Point-of-care testing in pharmacies–An evaluation of the service from the lens of resource-based theory of competitive advantage. *J Am Pharm Assoc.* 2021;61(2):e45–e54.
5. Rodis JL, Thomas RA. Stepwise approach to developing point-of-care testing services in the community/ambulatory pharmacy setting. *J Am Pharm Assoc.* 2006;46(5):594–604. doi:10.1331/1544-3191.46.5.594.rodis
6. Duquesne University. What is Business Model Canvas? Pittsburgh, PA: Duquesne University. Available at: https://www.sbdc.duq.edu/Blog-Item-What-is-Business-Model-Canvas. Accessed February 11, 2024.
7. United States Department of Labor. Occupational Safety and Health Administration. Training. Available at: https://www.osha.gov/training. Accessed February 11, 2024.
8. Hardin R, Roberts P, Hudspeth B, et al. Development and Implementation of an Influenza Point-Of-Care Testing Service in a Chain Community Pharmacy Setting. *Pharmacy*. 2020 Oct 6;8(4):182. doi:10.3390/pharmacy8040182
9. Houle S, Grindrod K, Chatterley T, et al. Paying pharmacists for patient care. *Can Pharm J.* 2014 Jul;147(4):209–232.
10. Bright D, Klepser M, Kelpser D. Pharmacist-provided point-of-care testing consultation service: a time and motion study. *J Pharm Tech*. 2018;34(4):139–143.
11. American Pharmacist Association. Billing Primer: A Pharmacist Guide to Outpatient Fee-for-Service Billing. Washington, DC: APhA. Available at: https://aphanet.pharmacist.com/sites/default/files/resource/APhABillingPrimer.pdf. Accessed February 11, 2024.
12. Hohmeier KC, Loomis B, Gatwood J. Consumer perceptions of and willingness-to-pay for point-of-care testing services in the community pharmacy. *Res Soc Admin Pharm*. 2018 Apr 1;14(4):360–366.

SECTION 2
Patient Care through Point-of-Care Testing and Treatment

CHAPTER 5

Patient Assessment and Point-of-Care Testing

Teresa E. Roane, PharmD, MBA, BCACP, CPh

Key Points

- POCT services offered in a community pharmacy setting improve patient care by increasing the pharmacist's accessibility to the patient.
- Pharmacy school curricula equip pharmacists with skills necessary for providing direct patient care services using established frameworks such as the Pharmacist Patient Care Process.
- A patient work-up should include a physical exam and vital sign assessment, as related to the patient's chief complaint, when providing POCT services.
- Creating and following policies and procedures help maintain good laboratory practices when providing POCT services.

Introduction

Over the past several years, pharmacy practice, particularly in the community-based setting, has seen an increase in pharmacists providing direct patient care services such as immunizations and POCT, as pharmacists have become more accessible for patients.[1-6] Several states have passed legislature allowing pharmacists (while working under an established protocol with other health care providers) to perform POCTs and then subsequently prescribe medications for patients for the treatment of minor non-chronic health conditions.[5,7-11] For some patients, community-based pharmacist-provided POCT services may be the patient's only option for care, as many patients do not have an established relationship with a primary care provider (PCP) and the pharmacist-provided services can occur outside of normal physician working hours.[6] With this added responsibility for pharmacists, it is important that they are equipped with the skills necessary for performing these expanded patient care services. This chapter covers the skills needed when conducting POCT services in the community-based pharmacy setting, including performing a patient work-up with corresponding physical assessment, following policies and procedures to ensure good laboratory practices when performing and analyzing POCTs, identifying basic processes and proper techniques for collecting the specimen to be tested, and establishing parameters and timeframes for following up with the patient after the initial encounter.

Patient Assessment

Although patient assessment skills are part of standards of education for pharmacy school curriculum (ACPE), not all practicing community-based pharmacists have been taught these skills, routinely utilize these skills, or feel comfortable in their ability to incorporate these skills into their practice, so it is important that they are a focus of the POCT training programs.[11-14] Patient assessment, for this chapter, will be divided into two different sections: communicating with the patient to determine the signs and symptoms the patient is experiencing that would preclude performing a POCT, and the subsequent physical assessment activities that correspond with evaluating the patient fully. Strategies for documenting the findings from the patient assessment and establishing a patient-centered follow-up plan will also be covered.

Patient Assessment: Communication Tools

In performing patient assessments, utilizing a systematic approach and consistent communication efforts provides for a better comprehensive approach to patient care.[15] There are a number of methods in practice; however, those covered in this chapter will include the Pharmacists' Patient Care Process (PPCP) and SCHOLAR-MAC,[15,16] a mnemonic for Symptoms, Characteristics, History, Onset, Location, Aggravating Factors, Remitting Factors, Medications, Allergies, and Coexisting Conditions.

The PPCP is recognized as a standard and consistent process for providing patient care services regardless of the pharmacists' practice setting.[15] The PPCP can be utilized in the community-based setting to help pharmacists evaluate a patient's symptoms and determine the feasibility of treating those symptoms for minor non-chronic health conditions. The PPCP is a continual process and the steps involved include: Collect, Assess, Plan, Implement, and Follow-up: Monitor and Evaluate.[15] Here is a brief overview of each of the steps in the process:

- In the Collect stage, the pharmacist uses their communication skills to talk with the patient to gather subjective information (reported by the patient) such as their chief complaint or the history of the present illness, including the symptoms the patient is currently experiencing.15 Objective data (obtained from patient records, diagnostic reports, and physical exam) are also gathered during this stage. Information about medications the patient is currently taking for any of their health conditions (chronic and non-chronic) is also collected.15 Also during the collect stage, the pharmacist performs any POCTs. POCT is performed outside of a laboratory setting and is commonly used in helping manage certain chronic conditions, such as testing blood glucose levels in patients with diabetes or international normalized ratio (INR) levels in patients taking blood thinners.15 These tests offer quick results and may be performed either by an HCP or the patient, depending on the type of test and health condition. POCTs performed by pharmacists offering test-and-treat services may be necessary to help confirm or rule out a non-chronic health condition suspected from gathering (and assessing) the patient's information and chief complaint or symptomology. Although the POCT step is part of the collect phase, it should occur after completing the patient work-up and physical exam elements to determine if testing is appropriate.

- In the Assess stage, the pharmacist reviews the information collected from the patient and the patient records to determine the appropriateness of current therapy and ensure that the patient is not having any issues related to their chronic therapy.[15] In addition, the results from the physical exam and the POCT performed (if performed) are assessed to determine the feasibility and appropriateness of adding a new medication for the patient's current symptoms.

- In the Plan stage, the pharmacist creates a patient-specific plan to address any issues identified within the patient's overall medication regimen (if any) and to help resolve any symptoms currently bothering the patient.[15] The plan may include adding prescription or nonprescription therapy based upon the patient's symptomology and the corresponding POCT results. A clear concise plan should be based on current guidelines and achieve desired outcomes, and it should be created in collaboration with the patient.

- In the Implement stage, the pharmacist initiates therapy, if appropriate, and provides counseling and education to the patient about the medication or supportive therapy recommended if adding a new medication is not warranted.[15] Documentation concerning the aspects of the patient encounter is incorporated into this phase. There are many forms of documentation, and the appropriate form will depend on the software system being utilized; however, the elements documented typically outline four specific areas: subjective (information gathered from the patient), objective (data gathered from the patient's records, during a physical exam, and from diagnostic reports), assessment, and plan (or SOAP).[17] Another aspect of the implementation phase includes reporting information back to the patient's PCP as outlined in the established pharmacist/HCP protocol. In addition, during the implementation step, a plan for follow-up with the patient is established.

- In the Follow-up: Monitor and Evaluate phase, the pharmacist talks with the patient again to see how the patient is doing since their previous encounter.[15] The pharmacist monitors outcomes from the initial plan, determines if the patient has had resolution of their symptoms, and ensures that no unintended consequences have occurred as a result of the initial plan. The follow-up can take place in person or over-the-phone and at a time point relevant to the plan of therapy (i.e., one or two days after starting a new antibiotic). If the patient has not had symptom resolution or experiences progression of symptoms, the pharmacist would repeat the process of collecting information from the patient and assessing that information to devise a new plan or consider a medical referral if necessary.

The PPCP is a good tool for consistently providing patient-centered care.

SCHOLAR-MAC is another type of communication tool that provides a framework to help pharmacists systematically assess a patient's current symptoms and the progression of that illness.[16] The SCHOLAR part of SCHOLAR-MAC focuses on the current symptoms the patient is experiencing and provides example questions for the pharmacist to ask of the patient.[16] The MAC portion of SCHOLAR-MAC incorporates an assessment of the patient's general medications to ensure that the pharmacist takes these medications into consideration when recommending treatment for the new condition.[16] The use of the SCHOLAR-MAC tool is also relevant when assessing patients for minor non-chronic health conditions regardless of the availability of a POCT for that suspected condition, such as when talking with a patient complaining of symptoms of mild acne, a cough, or head lice. The various characteristics of the SCHOLAR-MAC tool and example assessment questions are outlined in Table 5–1.[16]

Physical Assessment Activities

In addition to talking with the patient, elements of a physical exam should be incorporated into the encounter during POCT services to appropriately assess the patient and determine a plan of action for resolving complaints related to minor non-chronic health conditions.[15,19,20] These elements of the physical exam will vary depending on the patient's chief complaint and their associated symptoms, although it should always include an examination of general appearance and monitoring of vital signs related to symptomology.

Table 5–1. Elements of the SCHOLAR-MAC framework[16]

Element	Associated questions and assessment factors
Symptoms	What are the symptoms you are having right now?
Characteristics	How would you describe the symptoms (what are they like)?
History	Have you had these symptoms before? What have you taken for your symptoms?
Onset	When did the symptoms start (how long have you had these symptoms)?
Location	Where do you feel symptoms (i.e. nose, chest, throat, stomach)?
Aggravating factors	What do you feel makes the symptoms worse?
Remitting factors	What do you feel makes the symptoms better?
Medications	What medications are you currently taking (prescription, over-the-counter, supplements, etc.)?
Allergies	What medication allergies do you have? What reaction did you have to this medication?
Conditions	What medical conditions do you have (have you been diagnosed with)?

For a general appearance exam, the pharmacist should examine the patient's physical characteristics, including age, height, weight, gender, race, body type and build, and overall state of health (or sickness). In addition, the pharmacist should determine the patient's level of alertness (awake, attentive, and cooperative versus fatigued or lethargic).[19,20] The pharmacist should also consider the patient's state of comfort or distress. Is the patient experiencing noticeable pain or severe symptoms that would warrant a medical referral, or would it be feasible to continue to provide the POCT services in the community-based setting?

Vital sign assessment should be patient-centered and align with the patient's overall chief complaint; therefore, not all vital signs should be assessed for every patient. Vital signs and physical characteristics (other than those previously mentioned) the pharmacist should be familiar with and comfortable checking include body temperature, blood pressure, pulse, respiratory rate, and pulse oximetry, as well as lymph node palpation, a visual throat exam, the skin turgor test, and head hair examination for head lice.[19,20] In addition, the pharmacists should have confidence in listening to the patient's lungs and assessing breathing patterns and how they may differentiate from normal during times of distress.[19,20] Including these physical exam elements into POCT services will help guide prescribing options if the addition of medication therapy is warranted. POCT training programs, such as the American Pharmacists Association (APhA) Pharmacy-Based Test-and-Treat Program and the National Alliance of State Pharmacy Associations (NASPA) Pharmacy-Based Point-of-Care Test & Treat National Certificate Program,[21,22] incorporate specific details on how to perform the physical exam and vital sign assessment during the self-study content, which can help pharmacists gain proficiency and confidence in assessing these specific areas during a patient encounter. It is important to note that regulations for pharmacists providing patient care services, including physical assessment, may vary by state; therefore, it is important that the CPA or protocol document created outlines the pharmacists' responsibility for performing such services as delegated by the physician or the protocol.[23] Key points about each of the vital signs and physical characteristics mentioned above are included in Table 5–2.

Utilizing Good Laboratory Practices in the Community-Based Setting

Elements for establishing appropriate POCT services within the community-based pharmacy are covered in detail in Chapters 1–3. POCTs for chronic health conditions, such as blood glucose testing for diabetes, have long been established as common practices for pharmacists; however, pharmacists providing POCT services for minor non-chronic health conditions is a relatively new concept and only a few states allow pharmacists to perform such services.[4,5,7] It is the pharmacist's responsibility to ensure the use of best practices when administering POCT and interpreting the results. Best practices include following established policies and procedures for preparing and maintaining the testing site, collecting the specimen or sample, testing the sample collected, recording the results, and reporting the results.[17,24] The Centers for Disease Control and Prevention (CDC)'s booklet "Ready? Set? Test!" is a useful guide that can assist pharmacists throughout this process.[24] A brief overview of each section of this booklet and key points to consider when establishing a POCT program are described below.

Table 5-2. Clinical pearls for vital signs and physical exam characteristics[19,20]

Vital sign or physical examination	Clinical pearls
Body temperature	Temperature is measured with a thermometer (orally, rectally, axillary, or forehead); location of measurement can cause temperature to be lower/higher; normal body temperature is 97–99° F (for most people); temperature can fluctuate with time of day, based on physical exertion or stress, or when taking certain medications, drugs, or tobacco use
Blood pressure	Blood pressure (BP) is measured using a blood pressure monitor; use correct size cuff for patient's arm; proper positioning matters—have patient seated with arm supported and feet flat on the ground after resting for a few minutes; avoid conversation during blood pressure monitoring; ensure patient has an empty bladder prior to taking blood pressure
Pulse	Check pulse by feeling the radial artery in the inside of the patient's wrist using two fingers; resting pulse rate is ~60–100 beats per minute but can vary from minute to minute and patient to patient; avoid using the thumb to measure pulse; pulse can be higher when patient is hot, stressed, standing, or obese
Respiratory rate	Check respiratory rate (RR) by watching the patient breath; normal rate is ~12–16 breaths per minute; count breaths when patient is unaware as breathing can change if patient knows they are being watched; rate can be affected by alcohol and certain health conditions
Pulse oximetry	Pulse oximetry (PO) is measured using a pulse oximeter; measures the amount of oxygen saturation in the body; normal range is 95–100%; can be affected by bright light, poor circulation, skin pigment or thickness, nail polish, or current tobacco use
Lymph node palpation (head/ neck area)	Enlarged lymph nodes can be a sign of infection; most pharmacists are not comfortable assessing patient's lymph nodes but the test is easily performed; let patient know before touching them; evaluate for symmetry using two or three fingers, moving in a circular motion, lightly touching and applying gentle pressure to the patients lymph nodes; move from spot to spot in a systematic way comparing size and shape of lymph nodes while assessing for pain or tenderness
Visual throat exam	Examine mouth and throat using a bright light and tongue depressor; look for any abnormalities, redness, or white spots; expect patient to gag when applying pressure on the tongue with depressor or conducting throat swab test; have patient say "ahhh" to open up throat for better view
Skin turgor test	Also called the dehydration pinch test; let patient know before touching them; pinch a small area of skin on the top of the hand, pull it up, then release and measure the time to return to normal; also assess skin color, temperature, and moisture level
Hair examination (for head lice)	Use gloves to part patient's hair so scalp can be seen; systematically check sections of the hair, looking for live lice or their eggs (nits); nits are small and white/ light brown; nits are often found on the hair shaft or close to the scalp; nits are attached and do not normally slide up/down hair shaft; empty egg cases may appear white (meaning eggs have hatched and indicating a longer time of infestation); lice and/or nits are more often found in hair at the nape of neck or behind ears
Breath sounds/ listening to lungs	Ask patient to breathe in deeply; use stethoscope to listen to lungs/breath sounds; listen from front and back; move side to side and top to bottom while comparing lung sounds at each level; need to be familiar with normal and abnormal sounds

Prepare for testing

An area within the pharmacy should be designated specifically for POCT services.[24] The area should be clean, well lit, and contain appropriate testing supplies and materials, which may vary depending on the types of tests in the inventory. Supplies and materials may include a refrigerator, thermometer, timer, sufficient workspace, personal protective equipment, testing kits, bandages, sharps container, waste receptacle, hazardous waste collection bin, cleaning supplies, and a documentation system. An inventory of testing supplies and materials, along with the manufacturer instructions and storage requirements, should also be housed in this area. On a routine basis, the inventory should be checked to ensure that test kits are in date and ample supplies are on hand for providing testing services.

Getting ready for specimen collection

Prior to administering a POCT, always check the expiration date and review the manufacturer's full testing instructions.[24] The test components and instructions may change from lot to lot so this step should not be avoided. Become familiar with the components of the test kit, steps to take when administering the test, and when test results should be read. Also recognize what quality control mechanism is in place for each test kit in the inventory, because the quality control piece helps ensure that the test kit performs as intended. For some types of test kits, it is advisable to maintain a quality control log to record the steps conducted during the quality control assessment, the outcome of the quality control test, the test kit information with expiration date, and the person conducting the testing. In some cases, the quality control check is included as part of the testing process, so separate quality control checks may not be necessary. Specific requirements for quality control assessment are included in the product information for each test. Once these steps have been taken, the sample for testing can be collected.

Specimen collection

After it has been determined that a POCT should be performed on a patient, several steps should be performed during the specimen collection process.[24] First, determine the type of test to be conducted and what type of sample needs to be collected (e.g., blood, saliva, oropharyngeal, nasopharyngeal). Next, gather all of the appropriate supplies needed to administer the test. Verify the patient's information to ensure that the correct test kit is being used for the right patient. At this time, inform the patient about the steps necessary to conduct the test and how long it will take to receive the test results, and answer questions they may have about the test itself. Ensure that standard precautions are taken and safety guidelines are being followed, and put on appropriate PPE such as a mask, gloves, eye protection, a laboratory coat, and a gown. Finally, follow the manufacturer's specific instructions for the type and amount of sample needed to perform the test, because these requirements are likely to differ for each POCT kit.

Testing the sample

The manufacturer's instructions should be closely followed to determine the type and volume of sample needed, as well as the processing time required to complete the test.24

To collect a blood sample, ask the patient their preferred location for taking the sample (which fingertip or which arm), clean the area with an alcohol pad and let it dry, use an appropriate device to puncture the skin, wipe away the first drop of blood with a gauze pad, apply the blood droplet to the test strip or fill the capillary tube with the blood sample, place the sample in the testing machine, and then place a bandage on the patient's skin. For test kits that require samples from the nose or throat, determine the appropriate swab type (oropharyngeal or nasopharyngeal).

To collect a sample from the nose, have the patient tilt their head back slightly. Insert the swab through the patient's nares parallel to their palate, continue inserting the swab until resistance is encountered, gently rub and roll the swab around a few times in a circular motion, remove the swab, and then place the swab in the testing device. Some test kits may only require a swab from just inside the nostril, while others require sampling an area deeper inside.

To collect a sample from the throat, have the patient tilt their head back slightly, open their mouth wide, and say "ahhh." Use a tongue depressor to place pressure on the patient's tongue while simultaneously inserting the swab into the back of the throat. Gently rub the swab over both tonsillar pillars and the posterior oropharynx (avoiding the patient's teeth, tongue, and gums), remove the tongue depressor and throat swab, and place the swab sample into the testing device. Be prepared for the patient to gag during this test; consider standing to the left of the patient, rather than directly in front. Also consider having a trash can nearby in case the patient's gag reflux leads to vomiting.

To collect an oral fluid sample, place the sample collector into the patient's mouth and have the patient direct the saliva toward the collection pad. The collection technique and amount of oral fluid required may vary depending on the test. Instruct the patient to pool saliva in their mouth for a short period of time without swallowing. Alternatively, the patient may be instructed to spit saliva into the collection tube until the sample reaches a predetermined volume mark. Finally, the sample is placed into the testing device. Patients may find it difficult to collect sufficient saliva for a test sample, so additional time may be required to collect such samples.

Reading the results

Some test kits provide immediate results, while others are delayed.[24,25] The manufacturer's instructions will clearly state the time required to process the sample and obtain test results. Reading the results too soon can cause invalid or false negative results due to incomplete reaction of the sample and the components of the testing device. Reading the test results too long after the recommended interval can lead to false positive results due to over-development of color, false negative results due to fading of the reaction or color, or invalid results due to the reaction moving beyond the visible testing area. It is recommended to use a timer and follow the required timing intervals when reading the test results. The results will be displayed quantitatively, qualitatively, or as a combination of both types of results. Quantitative results are numbers produced by the test device and give the amount of the substance being measured in specific measurement units (e.g., for blood glucose results where the corresponding number is 140 mg/dL). Qualitative results are interpreted as positive, negative, reactive, non-reactive, or invalid (e.g., positive for influenza, negative for strep throat).

When interpreting test results, HCPs should consider the accuracy of the test, as well as the performance of the test for detecting the absence or presence of a condition. No test is 100% accurate, so most test kits contain documentation including values for sensitivity and specificity, which are both reported as a percentage.[26] The sensitivity of a test indicates how well the test correctly identifies the presence of a disease or condition. Sensitivity is associated with the tendency for a test to produce true positive or false negative results. When the sensitivity value is high, the test is more likely to accurately detect a true positive result. If a test has low sensitivity, the test is more likely to produce a high rate of false negative results, which indicate falsely that an afflicted patient does not have the condition being assayed. The specificity of a test indicates its capability to accurately detect the absence of a disease or condition. Specificity is associated with the tendency for a test to produce true negative or false positive results. A test with high specificity is more likely to yield a negative result for a patient that is not afflicted with the condition being assayed, while a test with low specificity is more likely to yield a positive result for a patient that does not have the condition. Sensitivity and specificity are important considerations during the process of choosing a test kit.

Documenting the results[24]

Logbooks or electronic files should be used to maintain records. The results of each test conducted should be documented as indicated in the pharmacy's policies and procedures. If electronic documentation is not feasible, ensure that handwritten results are legible. Quantitative results should be recorded using the appropriate units of measurement. Qualitative results should be recorded using words or abbreviations rather than symbols (i.e., "positive" or "pos" or "negative" or "neg" vs. "+" or "–"). Invalid or unacceptable results should also be recorded. If a test needs to be repeated, record the first result (invalid or unacceptable), resolve the problem, repeat the test, and then record the repeated result(s). In addition to the test results, document the recommended treatment plan for either positive or negative results.

After the Encounter: Follow-Up

The timeframe and format for follow-up care depend upon the patient, their chief complaint, and the pharmacist's plan of action. The follow-up assessment can take place in person or remotely and should occur at a time point relevant to the plan of therapy (e.g., 1 or 2 days after starting a new antibiotic). If the patient has not had symptom resolution or experiences progression of symptoms, the pharmacist should repeat the process of collecting information from the patient and assessing that information to devise a new plan of action or consider a medical referral if necessary.

Documentation Considerations

As previously mentioned, documentation is an important part of the process when providing patient care services, including POCT activities.[3,17] The format of the documentation may vary depending on the computer system or platform being utilized in the pharmacy setting, although the elements included from the encounter should not. Items to document include information collected from the patient interaction, findings from the physical assessment, results of the POCT activities if performed, the pharmacist's assessment of the situation, the plan for resolving the patient's chief complaint, and the plan for following up with the patient. It is good practice to develop and follow procedures, or even create templates, to ensure that required elements are consistently performed and documented for each patient encounter.[10] Documentation provides proof that services were conducted, allows for continuity of care at follow-up visits or should staffing changes occur, supports clinical activities should legal issues arise, and verifies activities performed for billing of the services (if allowed).[10] Only a few states currently allow pharmacists to provide POCT, and few of these states outline mechanisms by which pharmacists may be paid for such services.[7,22,26] Pharmacists are not considered providers according to Medicare, and other health insurance payers often follow suit with Medicare; therefore, pharmacists may not be allowed to bill insurance payers directly and may need to find other means of billing for patient care services, such as billing under a physician using incident-to billing codes.[4,26] Due to this billing inconsistency, the primary form of compensation for pharmacist-provided POCT services in the community setting is self-pay from the patient.

Example Patient Case

JT is a 21-year-old woman that comes into the pharmacy and approaches the pharmacy counter asking for the pharmacist. She says to the pharmacist, "I've started having this burning sensation when I go to the bathroom, and it hurts. Is there anything I can take for this?" The pharmacist responds, "That must be really uncomfortable for you. May I ask you some questions first so I can provide the best recommendation for you?" JT replies, "Yes."

Using SCHOLAR-MAC, the pharmacist collects the following information:

Element	Pharmacist's question	Patient's reply
Symptoms	"So, you are having a burning sensation when you go to the bathroom and say that 'it hurts.' Where does it hurt? What other symptoms are you having?"	"Yes, it hurts when I go pee. I feel a burning sensation and feel like I have to go pee, but then hardly anything comes out."
Characteristics	"So just the burning sensation and feeling of urgency with not a lot of pee coming out. How bad would you say it hurts on a scale of 1–10 with 10 being the worst pain? Describe the hurting or pain that you feel."	"I would say it hurts only when I try to go pee. It really is just a burning feeling. I would say a three out of 10 just walking around, but a seven out of 10 when I try to pee."
History	"Have you had these symptoms before? What have you taken for your symptoms?"	"No, I have never had this happen before. My mom told me to try drinking lots of water and some cranberry juice, but that doesn't seem to be helping!"
Onset	"When did the symptoms start (how long have you had these symptoms)"?	"This started just a couple of days ago; maybe 2 days ago."
Location	"Where do you feel symptoms? Just when you pee or is your back hurting also?"	"No, my back doesn't really hurt; just the burning feeling when I go to the bathroom."
Aggravating factors	"What do you feel makes the symptoms worse?" "Do you take bubble baths or use scented body wash?"	"Just having to go pee. I dread trying to go pee right now." "Now that you mention it, I did have a bubble bath a few days ago."
Remitting factors	"What do you feel makes the symptoms better?"	"It seems like a hot shower makes me feel better, but not much else does. Can you recommend something for me?"
Medications	"What medications are you currently taking (prescription, over-the-counter, supplements, etc.)? What health insurance coverage do you have, if any?"	"I do take a birth control pill every day but nothing else. I do not currently have any insurance."
Allergies	"What medication allergies do you have? What reaction did you have to this medication?"	"I am allergic to sulfa drugs. They cause me to break out into a rash."
Conditions	"What medical conditions do you have (have you been diagnosed with)?"	"None."

Example Patient Case 5-1 SOAP Note

Collect	Chief complaint (CC)
Subjective	Patient presents with burning sensation when urinating; patient is asking for medication
	History of present illness (HPI)
	21-year-old woman complaining of burning upon urination for 2 days
	Describes pain level as 7/10 when urinating and 3/10 otherwise; recent bubble bath exposure
Objective	Past medical history (PMH): unremarkable
	Medications: Seasonale (levonorgestrel/ethinyl estradiol tablets) 1 tablet daily
	Allergies: sulfa drugs (rash)
	Height: 63 in; weight: 115 lbs; BP: 114/78; P: 78; RR: 16
Assess	Based on the information gathered from the patient, it is likely that she is experiencing a urinary tract infection (UTI). This may have been precipitated by a recent bubble bath.
Plan	A point-of-care urine dipstick test could be performed; however, currently available POCT tests for UTI are for patient self-use and not very practical in the pharmacy setting. In addition, such tests would be unlikely to change the treatment recommendations. Treatment options for UTI for this patient include nitrofurantoin 100 mg twice daily for 5 days, sulfamethoxazole/trimethoprim 800/160 mg twice daily for 3 days, or fosfomycin 3 gm taken as one single dose. Due to the patient having a sulfa allergy, her options include nitrofurantoin or fosfomycin. Of these two options, fosfomycin is likely more expensive. Given that the patient does not have health insurance, recommend nitrofurantoin 100 mg twice daily for 5 days.
Implement	Start nitrofurantoin 100 mg: take 1 capsule by mouth twice daily for 5 days. Counsel patient: this medication may cause upset stomach so recommend taking it with food to help minimize this adverse effect. It is important to not miss any doses and take the full 5-day course of this medicine. Also start Azo Urinary Pain Relief: take 2 tablets by mouth three times daily for up to 2 days to help with the burning sensation. Counsel patient: this medication does not cure a urinary tract infection. It may also cause urine discoloration, so it is important to educate the patient about this effect as well.
Monitor/ Follow-up	Follow-up with the patient by phone within 24–48 hours to determine if she is having any symptom relief, if she is experiencing any adverse effects from the antibiotic, or if her symptoms have progressed.

Conclusion

When a patient approaches with a chief complaint and seeks symptom relief, accurately conducting the patient assessment determines if POCT is appropriate. Communicating with the patient in a systematic way using a standard format, such as SCHOLAR-MAC, and incorporating the appropriate physical assessment techniques helps the pharmacist gather the necessary information to formulate an appropriate plan for treatment and follow-up care. If POCT is warranted, utilizing good laboratory practices ensures that quality results are obtained, which can guide recommendations for appropriate patient care.

References

1. Urick BY, Meggs EV. Towards a Greater Professional Standing: Evolution of Pharmacy Practice and Education, 1920–2020. *Pharmacy (Basel)*. 2019; 7(3):98. Published 2019 Jul 20. doi:10.3390/pharmacy7030098

2. Klepser DG, Klepser ME. Point-of-care testing in the pharmacy: how is the field evolving? *Expert Rev Mol Diagn*. 2018;18(1):5–6. doi:10.1080/14737159.2018.1392240

3. Gutierres SL, Welty TE. Point-of-care testing: an introduction. *Ann Pharmacother*. 2004;38(1):119–125. doi:10.1345/aph.1D212

4. Goode JV, Owen J, Page A, Gatewood S. Community-Based Pharmacy Practice Innovation and the Role of the Community-Based Pharmacist Practitioner in the United States. *Pharmacy (Basel)*. 2019;7(3):106. Published 2019 Aug 4. doi:10.3390/pharmacy7030106

5. Hardin R, Roberts P, Hudspeth B, et al. Development and implementation of an influenza point-of-care testing service in a chain community pharmacy setting. *Pharmacy (Basel)*. 2020;8(4):182. Published 2020 Oct 6. doi:10.3390/pharmacy8040182

6. Wolters Kluwer. Pharmacy Next: Consumer trends and industry transformation. Alphen aan den Rijn, the Netherlands: Wolters Kluwer. Available at: https://www.wolterskluwer.com/en/know/pharmacy-next?&utm_medium=press_release&utm_source_web&utm_campaign=pharmacynext_awareness_pharmacynext_May2023. Accessed February 11, 2024.

7. Page A, Owen JA, Goode JR, Kuhn C, Skelton JB. Pharmacist-initiated treatment of minor conditions: A call to action. *J Am Pharm Assoc (2003)*. 2021; 61(1):13–19. doi:10.1016/j.japh.2020.09.021

8. Sachdev G, Kliethermes MA, Vernon V, Leal S, Crabtree G. Current status of prescriptive authority by pharmacists in the United States. *J Am Coll Clin Pharm*. 2020;3:807–817. doi:10.1002/jac5.1245

9. Gubbins PO, Klepser ME, Dering-Anderson AM, et al. Point-of-care testing for infectious diseases: Opportunities, barriers, and considerations in community pharmacy. *J Am Pharm Assoc (2003)*. 2014;54(2):163–171.doi:10.1331/JAPhA.2014.13167

10. Gallimore CE, Porter AL, Barnett SG, Portillo E, Zorek JA. A state-level needs analysis of community pharmacy point-of-care testing. *J Am Pharm Assoc (2003)*. 2021;61(3):e93–e98. doi:10.1016/j.japh.2020.12.013

11. Koski RR, Klepser N, Koski M, Klepser M, Klepser D. Community pharmacist-provided test and treat programs for acute infectious conditions. *J Am Coll Clin Pharm*. 2023;1–11. doi:10.1002/jac5.1793

12. Accreditation Council for Pharmacy Education. Accreditation standards and key elements for the professional program leading to the doctor of pharmacy degree. Standards 2016. Chicago, IL: ACPE. Available at: https://www.acpe-accredit.org/pdf/Standards2016FINAL.pdf. Accessed February 11, 2024.

13. Kehrer JP, James DE. The Role of Pharmacists and Pharmacy Education in Point-of-Care Testing. *Am J Pharm Educ*. 2016;80(8):129. doi:10.5688/ajpe808129

14. McKeirnan K, Czapinski J, Bertsch T, Buchman C, Akers J. Training Student Pharmacists to Perform Point-of-Care Testing. *Am J Pharm Educ*. 2019; 83(7):7031. doi:10.5688/ajpe7031

15. Joint Commission of Pharmacy Practitioners (JCPP). Pharmacists' Patient Care Process. Alexandria, VA: JCPP. Available at: https://jcpp.net/wp-content/uploads/2016/03/PatientCareProcess-with-supporting-organizations.pdf. Accessed February 11, 2024.

16. Buring SM, Kirby J, Conrad WF. A structured approach for teaching students to counsel self-care patients. *Am J Pharm Educ*. 2007;71(1):8. doi: 10.5688/aj710108

17. Rodis JL, Thomas RA. Stepwise approach to developing point-of-care testing services in the community/ambulatory pharmacy setting. *J Am Pharm Assoc (2003)*. 2006;46(5):594–604. doi:10.1331/1544-3191.46.5.594.rodis

18. Introduction to Patient Assessment for Pharmacists. In: Herrier RN, Apgar DA, Boyce RW, Foster SL, eds. *Patient Assessment in Pharmacy*. McGraw Hill; 2015. Available at: https://accesspharmacy.mhmedical.com/content.aspx?bookid=1074&sectionid=62363577. Accessed February 11, 2024.

19. Bello-Quintero CE, Bardowell RH. Chapter 10. Physical Assessment Skills. In: Nemire RE, Kier KL, eds. *Pharmacy Student Survival Guide*, 2e. McGraw Hill; 2009. Available at: https://accesspharmacy.mhmedical.com/content.aspx?bookid=512&sectionid=41742439. Accessed February 11, 2024.

20. Leong C, Soufi L. Physical assessment in pharmacy practice: Perspectives from pharmacists, nonpharmacist health care providers and the public. *Can Pharm J* (Ott). 2021;154(3):193–204. Published 2021 Apr 21. doi:10.1177/17151635211004975

21. American Pharmacists Association. Pharmacy-based Test and Treat Certificate Training Program. Washington, DC: APhA. Available at: https://www.pharmacist.com/Education/Certificate-Training-Programs/Pharmacy-Based-Test-And-Treat. Accessed February 11, 2024.

22. National Alliance of State Pharmacy Associations. NASPA Pharmacy-Based Point-of-Care Test & Treat National Certificate Program. Richmond, VA: NASPA. Available at: https://naspa.us/resource/pharmacy-based-point-of-care-testing-certification-program/. Accessed February 11, 2024.

23. Centers for Disease Control and Prevention. Collaborative Practice Agreements and Pharmacists' Patient Care Services: A Resource for Pharmacists. Atlanta, GA: CDC. Available at: https://www.cdc.gov/dhdsp/pubs/docs/translational_tools_pharmacists.pdf. Accessed February 11, 2024.

24. Centers for Disease Control and Prevention. Ready? Set? Test! Booklet: Patient Testing is Important. Get the right results. Atlanta, GA: CDC. Available at: https://www.cdc.gov/labquality/waived-tests.html. Accessed February 11, 2024.

25. National Council for Prescription Drug Programs, Inc. Billing Guidance for Pharmacists' Professional and Patient Care Services: V2.0. Scottsdale, AZ: NCPDP. Available at: https://www.ncpdp.org/NCPDP/media/pdf/WhitePaper/Billing-Guidance-for-Pharmacists-Professional-and-Patient-Care-Services-White-Paper.pdf. Accessed February 11, 2024.

26. Centers for Disease Control and Prevention. Diagnostic Sensitivity and Specificity for Clinical Laboratory Testing. Atlanta, GA: CDC. Available at: https://www.cdc.gov/labtraining/docs/job_aids/additional_resources/Sensitivity_and_Specificity_Final_5_23_2022_508.pdf. Accessed February 11, 2024.

CHAPTER 6

Influenza

Jeffrey Hamper, PharmD, BCACP

Key Points

- Influenza is a viral infection that has resulted in 9–41 million illnesses, 140,000–710,000 hospitalizations, and 12,000–52,000 deaths annually in the United States from 2010–2020.
- Influenza diagnosis may be made based on symptoms or testing, depending on the patient's symptoms, care setting, and influenza activity in the local community.
- POCTs for influenza include molecular assays that detect viral RNA or nucleic acids, and RIDTs that detect influenza antigens.
- Timely diagnosis of influenza may decrease unnecessary laboratory testing for other causes, may decrease the use of antibiotics, may improve the effectiveness of infection control and prevention measures, and may increase appropriate use of antiviral medications.
- Four antiviral medications (baloxavir, oseltamivir, peramivir, and zanamivir) are FDA-approved for prevention and treatment of influenza and may reduce symptom duration and severity of disease.

Influenza, commonly referred to as flu, is a viral infection caused by the influenza virus. The influenza virus is a single-stranded RNA virus from the orthomyxovirus family.[1] Of the four types of influenza viruses, A, B, and C are known to affect humans. The surface antigens hemagglutinin (HA) and neuraminidase (NA) determine the 18 different H subtypes, and 11 different N subtypes, of influenza A. Influenza B is classified into lineages, rather than the subtype classifications used for influenza A. There are two lineages of influenza B, which are B/Yamagata and B/Victoria.[1]

Influenza A viruses are the only influenza viruses known to cause flu pandemics, or worldwide epidemics of influenza disease. Influenza B more commonly affects children, and influenza C is rarely reported as a cause of human illness and has not been associated with epidemic disease. Influenza D viruses primarily affect cattle, with spillover to other animals, but are not known to infect humans.[2] Influenza viruses undergo constant genetic changes that affect immunity and considerations for vaccine composition each year. These changes include antigenic drift via mechanisms such as point mutations and recombination events, and antigenic shifts, which are larger genetic change events.[3]

People throughout the world and of any age are susceptible to influenza.[1,3] The incidence of influenza has been estimated to be approximately 8% (varying from 3% to 11%), although the exact incidence is difficulty to determine, as those infected often do not seek medical attention or receive a diagnosis.[3] While the timing varies year to year, annual epidemics of influenza typically occur during fall and winter in the United States, with activity starting during October and peaking in winter. Between 1982 and 2018, peak influenza activity most often occurred in February (42%), but also peaked in December (19%), January (17%), and March (17%).[3]

From 2010–2020, CDC estimates that influenza resulted in 9 to 41 million illnesses, between 140,000–710,000 hospitalizations, and 12,000–52,000 deaths annually in the United States.[4] Increases in mortality typically occur during each influenza season from influenza and pneumonia, as well as cardiopulmonary and other chronic diseases that can be exacerbated by influenza. Racial and ethnic disparities have also been associated with severe flu-related outcomes, including hospitalization, ICU admission, and in-hospital death.[5] When adjusted for age, Black persons had the highest flu-associated hospitalization, followed by American Indian or Alaska Native and Hispanic persons, with similar trends for ICU admission rates.[5]

Clinical Presentation

Influenza is transmissible from the day before symptom onset to about 5–7 days after symptoms begin, and children can transmit influenza to others for more than 10 days after symptoms begin.[1] Symptoms may last for two to eight days, may vary from person to person, and are often confused with symptoms of the common cold.[6,7] Common symptoms of influenza are listed in Box 6–1, and a comparison of flu and cold symptoms is included in Table 6–1.[1,6,8]

Box 6-1. Signs and symptoms of influenza[1,6,8]

Abdominal pain, diarrhea, and/or vomiting
Fatigue or tiredness
Fever[a] and/or chills
Headaches
Malaise

Muscle or body aches
Nonproductive cough
Runny or stuffy nose
Sore throat/hoarseness

[a] Not all patients with influenza will present with fever.

Table 6-1. Comparison of symptoms between the common cold, influenza, and COVID-19[1,6,8,9]

Signs and symptoms	Cold	Flu	COVID-19
Symptom onset	Gradual	Typically appear 1 to 4 days after infection	May appear anywhere from 2 to 5 days, and up to 14 days after infection
Fever	Rare	Common, lasts 3 to 4 days	Common
Aches	Slight	Common, often severe	Common
Extreme exhaustion	Never	Usual, at the beginning of illness	Common
Fatigue, weakness	Sometimes	Usual	Common
Sneezing	Common	Sometimes	Rare
Chest discomfort	Mild to moderate	Common	Common; call for emergency care if persistent pain, pressure, or difficulty breathing
Cough	Hacking cough	Can be severe	Common, dry cough
Stuffy or runny nose	Common	Sometimes	Common
Sore throat	Common	Sometimes	Common
Headache	Rare	Common	Common
Loss of taste or smell	Rare	Rare	Common

Most patients will recover from flu in less than 2 weeks, but some may develop complications that can be life-threatening and may result in death.[6] Populations at the most risk of developing serious complications related to influenza include patients over the age of 65; people with chronic pulmonary, cardiovascular, renal, hepatic, hematologic, or metabolic conditions; neurologic and neurodevelopment conditions; persons with immunosuppression; pregnant women and young children (<5 years, and especially aged <2 years); American Indian/Alaska native people; persons with extreme obesity (BMI >40 kg/m2); and residents of nursing homes and other chronic care facilities.[8] Common and other less common complications of influenza are listed in Table 6-2.[1,6]

Table 6–2. Common and other less common complications of influenza[1,6]

Common	Other less common complications
Bronchitis	Aseptic meningitis
Exacerbations of underlying respiratory conditions	Encephalitis
Laryngotracheobronchitis, also known as croup	Guillain-Barré syndrome
Otitis media	Myocarditis
Secondary bacterial pneumonia	Pericarditis
	Primary pneumonia
	Reye's syndrome
	Transverse myelitis

People experiencing warning signs of flu should obtain medical care as soon as possible.[10] In adults, these warning signs include shortness of breath and difficulty breathing, pressure or persistent chest or abdomen pain, persistent dizziness, confusion, inability to arouse, seizures, not urinating, severe muscle pain, severe weakness, unsteadiness, fever or cough that improve but then return, or worsen and worsening of chronic medical conditions.

Diagnosis and Physical Assessment

Timely diagnosis of influenza may decrease unnecessary laboratory testing, may decrease unnecessary use of antibiotics, may improve the effectiveness of infection control and prevention, and may increase appropriate use of antiviral medications.[8] Recommendations for which patients should be tested vary by the setting and level of influenza activity in the local community.[7,8] A summary of recommendations in the outpatient setting is listed in Table 6–3.[7,8]

Table 6–3. Recommendations for which patients should be tested for influenza in the outpatient setting[a] (including emergency department patients)[7,8]

During influenza activity[b]	• Clinicians should test for influenza in high-risk patients who present with influenza-like illness if the result will influence clinical management. • Clinicians should test for influenza in patients who present with acute respiratory symptoms with or without fever, and either exacerbation of chronic medical conditions or known complications of influenza, if the testing will influence clinical management. • Clinicians can consider influenza testing for patients not at high risk for influenza complications who present with influenza-like illness and who are likely to be discharged home if the results might influence antiviral treatment decisions or reduce use of unnecessary antibiotics, further diagnostic testing, and time in the emergency department, or if the results might influence influenza antiviral treatment or chemoprophylaxis decisions for high-risk household contacts.
During low influenza activity, without any link to an influenza outbreak	• Clinicians can consider influenza testing in patients with acute onset of respiratory symptoms with or without fever, especially for immunocompromised and high-risk patients.

[a]For recommendations related to testing for hospitalized patients, refer to the Clinical Practice Guidelines by the Infectious Diseases Society of America: 2018 Update on Diagnosis, Treatment, Chemoprophylaxis, and Institutional Outbreak Management of Seasonal Influenza.
[b]Influenza activity is defined as the circulation of seasonal influenza A and B viruses among people in the local community.

Testing for influenza virus is not always necessary to start antiviral treatment in a patient with suspected influenza, especially when activity is high in the local community. In these situations, diagnosis may be made clinically based on signs and symptoms, or if the patient has a suspected influenza-associated complication such as exacerbation of a chronic disease.[7] A symptom-only prediction rule (Table 6–4) may be used to aid clinicians in diagnosing influenza.[7] With this tool, points are assigned based on the type and number of symptoms a patient displays. Patients with two or fewer points have a low risk for influenza, while patients with four or more points have a high risk and may be considered for empiric treatment.[7]

Table 6–4. Symptom-only clinical prediction rule for diagnosing influenza[7]

Symptoms	Points assigned[a]
Fever and cough	2 points
Myalgias	2 points
Chills or sweats	1 point
Onset of symptoms within the past 48 hours	1 point

[a]Patients with two or fewer points are at low risk of influenza. Patients with four or more points are at high risk and may be considered for empiric treatment.

Point-of-Care Testing

The currently available POCTs for detecting influenza in respiratory specimens include molecular assays and antigen detection tests. Molecular assay tests include rapid molecular assays, reverse transcriptase-polymerase chain reaction (RT-PCR), and other nucleic acid amplification tests, which work by identifying the presence of influenza viral RNA or nucleic acids in respiratory tract specimens. Antigen detection tests include rapid influenza diagnostic tests (RIDTs) and immunofluorescence assays.[8,11] RIDTs detect influenza A and B viral nucleoprotein antigens in respiratory specimens.[8] Immunofluorescence assays use a fluorescent microscope for antigen detection. Direct (DFA), and indirect fluorescent antibody (IFA) staining assays detect both influenza A and B antigens in respiratory tract specimens. RIDTs can produce results in as little as 15 minutes. Immunofluorescence assay-based tests are not currently CLIA-waived. Viral culture and serologic tests are also sometimes performed in institutional settings, but these tests are not used to inform clinical management as they do not produce timely results.[11] A summary of currently available CLIA-waived POCTs for influenza A and B is provided in Table 6–5.[8,11–13]

Table 6-5. CLIA-waived POCTs for influenza A and B[8,11-13]

Test method[a]	Mechanism	Example brands[b]	Sample type[d]	Sensitivity/ specificity	Time for result	Key points	Relative cost comparison ($, $$, $$$)
Rapid influenza molecular assays	Influenza viral RNA or nucleic acid detection	- Abbott ID Now - Biofire FilmArray - Cepheid Xpert Xpress - Mesa Accula Flu - Roche Cobas - Sekisui Silaris	Nasopharyngeal swab, nasal swab	Moderate to High (66–99%)/ High (55–99%)	15–30 minutes	IDSA recommends use of rapid influenza molecular assays over RIDTs for detection of influenza viruses in respiratory specimens of outpatients	$$
Rapid influenza diagnostic tests (RIDTs)	Antigen detection[c]	- Abbott Binax Now - BD Veritor - OraSure QuickFlu - Quidel QuickVue - Quidel Sofia - Sekisui Acucy - Sekisui OSOM Ultra	Nasopharyngeal swab, aspirate or wash, nasal swab, aspirate or wash, throat swab	Moderate (50–70%)[d]/ High (>90%)	10–15 minutes	May result in false negatives or positives depending on flu activity	$

Key: IDSA, Infectious Disease Society of America; RIDT, rapid influenza diagnostic test.
[a]Some, but not all, rapid influenza molecular assays and rapid influenza diagnostic tests are CLIA-waived for POCT use.
[b]Approved specimens vary by test. Refer to manufacturer's package insert for specific test information.
[c]Detection of influenza virus antigen does not necessarily indicate detection of viable infectious virus, or ongoing influenza viral replication.
[d]Results of some RIDTs may be improved to 75–80% sensitivity using an analyzer reader to standardize results. FDA now requires RIDTs to achieve 80% sensitivity.

To properly interpret influenza POCT results, clinicians should consider the context of influenza activity and the limitations of diagnostic tests with lower sensitivity to detect influenza.[8] Interpretation of results depends on multiple factors, including influenza activity within the community, pre-test probability, whether influenzas viruses are actively replicating or have recently infected the patient, the time from symptom onset to specimen collection, the source and quality of respiratory specimens, the characteristics of the test being used, and whether proper procedures were used for specimen collection, transport, and testing.[8] Table 6-6 provides information about the interpretation of positive and negative results for POCT influenza tests.[8,11]

Table 6-6. Interpretation of influenza POCTs[8,11]

Result	Influenza activity	Interpretation and key points
RIDT	High influenza activity	Positive result: Positive predictive value is high. • Likely to be a true positive result. • False positive results are less likely with RIDTs but do occur and are more common during periods of low influenza activity. • When interpreting RIDT results, clinicians should consider the test in the context of the level of influenza activity in their community.
		Negative result: Negative predictive value is low. • May be a false negative result, especially if upper respiratory tract specimen was collected >4 days after illness onset; cannot exclude influenza virus infection. • RIDTs with low-moderate sensitivity and high specificity may tend to produce false negative results, especially during peak influenza activity in the community. Clinicians should consider confirming negative test results with molecular assays, especially during peak flu activity and/or during institutional influenza outbreaks. • Do not withhold antiviral treatment if clinically indicated.
	Low influenza activity	Positive result: Positive predictive value is low. • Likely to be a false positive result. • Confirm with a molecular assay.
		Negative result: Negative predictive value is high. • Likely to be a true negative result if an upper respiratory tract specimen was collected <4 days after illness onset. • If epidemiologically linked to an influenza outbreak, consider confirming with a molecular assay.
Molecular assay	High influenza activity	Positive result: Positive predictive value is high. • Likely to be a true positive result.
		Negative result: Negative predictive value is low. • May be a true negative result in a patient without lower respiratory tract disease. • Consider the potential for false negative results.
	Low influenza activity	Positive result: Positive predictive value is low. • False positive results are possible.
		Negative result: Negative predictive value is high. • Very likely to be a true negative result. • Influenza virus infection is unlikely if specimen was collected <4 days after illness onset and there is no epidemiological link to an influenza outbreak or travel to areas where influenza viruses are circulating. Should still consider the potential for false negative results.

Key: RIDT, rapid influenza diagnostic test.

Point-of-Care Testing for Special Populations

RIDTs should not be used for testing patients with progressive illness, patients with high risk for influenza complications, or hospitalized patients with suspected influenza.[8] Molecular assays can be used for both outpatients and hospitalized patients, and

RT-PCR should be used for hospitalized patients.[8] Patients who receive a live attenuated influenza virus vaccine via intranasal administration can shed influenza virus vaccine strains in the upper respiratory tract for up to seven days after intranasal vaccination and can test positive during this period.[8] Positive test results do not exclude bacterial coinfection, and evaluation of the potential need for antibiotics, especially in patients with pneumonia, should be considered.[8]

Treatment

Many people with flu have mild illness and may not seek diagnosis and treatment. Those experiencing minor flu symptoms should stay home and rest, avoid contact with other people, stay hydrated, and treat symptoms when necessary (e.g., acetaminophen or ibuprofen for fever or pain).[9] Dosing information for over-the-counter fever and pain relief options are provided in Table 6–7.[14–16] Aspirin and other salicylate-containing over-the-counter treatments should be avoided in patients younger than 18 years old due to increased risk of Reye's syndrome.[9] Common complementary health approaches, such as herbal products, sinus rinses, vitamin C, and zinc have not been shown to be helpful for influenza.[17]

Table 6–7. Over-the-counter options for treatment of fever, pain, and myalgia symptoms of influenza[14–16]

Product	Common brand names	Adult over-the-counter dose	Counseling points
Acetaminophen	Tylenol	325 to 650 mg every 4 to 6 hours as needed or 1 g every 6 hours as needed	Maximum dose is 4 g/day. Lower doses may be considered when used for extended periods, or for patients with risk factors for hepatotoxicity.
Ibuprofen	Advil, Motrin	200 to 400 mg every 4 to 6 hours as needed	Maximum OTC dose is 1.2 g/day. Use for >3 days is not recommended unless directed by an HCP. Avoid or use with caution in patients at risk for, or with, existing cardiovascular disease, GI disease, kidney impairment, chronic liver disease, or increased bleeding.
Naproxen	Aleve	200 to 400 mg once, followed by 200 mg every 8 to 12 hours as needed	Maximum OTC dose is 400 mg in any 8- to 12-hour period or 600 mg in a 24-hour period. Use the lowest effective dose for the shortest possible duration of time. Avoid or use with caution in patients at risk for, or with, existing cardiovascular disease, GI disease, kidney impairment, chronic liver disease, or risk for increased bleeding. Naproxen is available as naproxen base and sodium salt. A 200 mg base is equivalent to 220 mg naproxen sodium.

Early treatment with antivirals reduces duration of symptoms, decreases the risk of some complications and hospitalizations, and may decrease mortality among high-risk populations. The main benefits of antiviral treatment for influenza are reduced disease severity and decreased symptom duration (approximately 24-hour reduction if initiated within 36 hours of symptom onset).[7]

Treatment recommendations are based on signs and symptoms, individual patient characteristics, and influenza test results, if applicable. A general testing and treatment approach with drug therapy recommendations is provided in Figure 6–1.[7,8,18] A summary of pharmacologic treatments is provided in Table 6–8.[7,8,18]

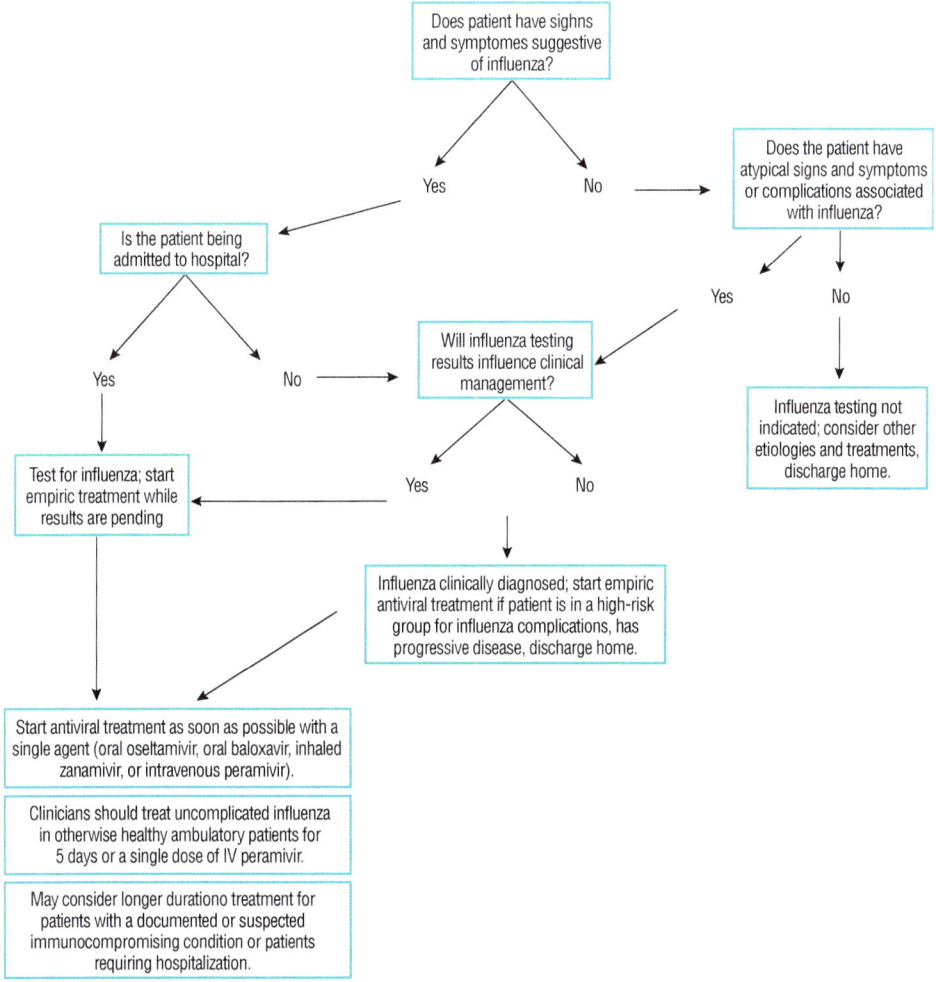

Figure 6–1. General testing and treatment approach for influenza[7,8,13]

Antiviral treatment should be initiated as soon as possible for patients with confirmed or suspected influenza, regardless of immunization status, who are either[8]:

- Patients of any age hospitalized with influenza, regardless of illness duration prior to hospitalization
- Outpatients with severe or progressive illness, regardless of illness duration
- Outpatients at risk of influenza complications, including immunocompromised patients and those with chronic medical conditions
- Children younger than two and adults over 65 years of age
- Pregnant women and patients within 2 weeks postpartum

Clinicians may consider antiviral treatment for adults who are not at high risk for influenza complications, with confirmed or suspected influenza, regardless of vaccination history, that meet any of the following criteria.[8]

- Outpatients with illness onset <2 days before presentation
- Symptomatic outpatients who are household contacts of someone at high risk of developing complications from influenza, particularly those who are severely immunocompromised
- Symptomatic HCPs who routinely care for patients at high risk of developing influenza complications, particularly those who are severely immunocompromised

If a patient with influenza does not demonstrate clinical improvement with antiviral treatment, or demonstrates clinical deterioration during or after treatment, the patient should be referred to investigate other causes besides influenza infection.[8]

Table 6-8. Pharmacologic agents for treatment and chemoprophylaxis of influenza[7,8,18]

Pharmacologic agent	Dose (treatment)	Dose (chemoprophylaxis)	Contraindications and precautions	Potential adverse effects
Oseltamivir (Tamiflu)[a]	Adults: 75 mg twice daily for 5 days Pregnancy: 75 mg twice daily for 5 days	Adults: 75 mg daily Pregnancy: 75 mg daily	Preferred agent for pregnant patients, and patients with severe influenza. Contraindicated in people with serious hypersensitivity to oseltamivir or any component of the product.	Nausea, vomiting, and allergic reactions such as rash and facial swelling.
Zanamivir (Relenza)	10 mg (two 5 mg inhalations) twice daily for 5 days	10 mg (two 5 mg inhalations) once daily	Caution should be used in patients with cognitive or physical limitations to ensure correct usage of inhaler device. Contraindicated in patients with milk allergy, underlying reactive airway disease (e.g., asthma, COPD), or history of allergic reaction to zanamivir or any component of the product. May use during pregnancy; risk of embryo-fetal toxicity not expected based on human data.	Headaches, diarrhea, nausea, vomiting, allergic reaction, nasal symptoms, bronchitis, cough, sinusitis, dizziness, fever, chills, arthralgia, and articular rheumatism. Serious and sometimes fatal cases of bronchospasm have occurred.
Peramivir (Rapivab)[a]	Adults: 600 mg intravenous infusion once, given over 15–30 minutes	N/A	Contraindicated in patients with serious hypersensitivity or anaphylaxis to peramivir or any component of the product.	Diarrhea, nausea, vomiting, and neutropenia
Baloxavir (Xofluza)	Adults: >80 kg: 80 mg as a single dose <80 kg: 40 mg as a single dose	Adults: >80 kg: 80 mg as a single dose <80 kg: 40 mg as a single dose	Contraindicated in those with a history of hypersensitivity to baloxavir or any component of the product. Avoid use in pregnancy.	Diarrhea, bronchitis, nasopharyngitis, headache, and nausea

Key: COPD, chronic obstructive pulmonary disease.
[a]Oseltamivir and peramivir doses must be adjusted for treatment or chemoprophylaxis in adults with renal impairment or end-stage renal disease on dialysis. See prescribing information for detailed dosage information. A longer duration can be considered in severely ill or immunocompromised patients.

Pharmacists in several states, including Arkansas, Colorado, Delaware, Idaho, Iowa, and Kansas, have direct prescriptive authority for the testing and treatment of flu, while other states, such as Florida and Kentucky, have delegated prescribing authority or may work under a CPA.[19] Scope of practice and criteria will vary by state, and pharmacists should contact their state board of pharmacy for current state-specific information. Some considerations for community-based pharmacists are listed in Table 6–9.[20-22]

Table 6–9. Considerations for community-based pharmacists regarding testing, treating, and managing influenza[20-22]

Can a pharmacist prescribe or dispense pharmacologic treatment for influenza based on POCT results under a collaborative practice agreement, standing order, or state protocol?	Considerations

Yes	• Consider referring patient for situations including, but not limited to:
	  • Patient does not meet eligibility criteria for a POCT
	  • Patient is indicated for confirmatory testing
	  • Patient is indicated for urgent or emergency care
	  • Patient has previously been prescribed influenza treatment with no improvement of symptoms
	  • Empiric treatment would be started by an HCP without testing
	• Consider educating patient on items such as:
	  • Importance of annual influenza vaccination
	  • Infection control measures
	  • Appropriate self-care measures and treatment of symptoms
	  • When to seek urgent or emergency care

No	• Consider referring patient for situations including, but not limited to:
	  • Patient meets eligibility criteria for influenza testing and treatment
	  • Patient is indicated for urgent or emergency care
	  • Patient has previously been prescribed influenza treatment with no improvement of symptoms
	  • Empiric treatment would be started by an HCP without testing
	• Consider educating patient on items such as:
	  • Importance of annual influenza vaccination
	  • Infection control measures
	  • Appropriate self-care measures and treatment of symptoms
	  • When to seek urgent or emergency care

Chemoprophylaxis

Vaccination is the preferred method for prevention of influenza, and the routine use of chemoprophylaxis against influenza is not recommended. However, chemoprophylaxis for the prevention of influenza may be used in specific populations. A summary of recommendations from the Infectious Disease Society of America (IDSA) for chemoprophylaxis of influenza in community settings is provided in Table 6–10.[7,8]

Table 6–10. Recommendations for chemoprophylaxis of influenza in community settings[7,8]

Indication for prophylaxis	Initiation	Duration
People at high risk of complications of influenza	Postexposure • Within 48 hours of initial exposure if unable to vaccinate or vaccine effectiveness is likely to be low after close contact exposure to a person with influenza	7 days after initial exposure
Use in conjunction with vaccination for unvaccinated people in close contact with a person at high risk of influenza complications	Postexposure • Within 48 hours of initial exposure to a person with influenza	At least 7 days after initial exposure or until vaccine effectiveness is likely achieved
Unvaccinated people at high risk of influenza complications	Postexposure • Within 48 hours of initial exposure in conjunction with vaccination after exposure to a person with influenza	14 days or until vaccine effectiveness is likely achieved
People at high risk of developing complications of influenza if unable to vaccinate or vaccine likely to be ineffective when influenza is present (immune deficiency)	Pre-exposure	Duration of influenza activity
People at the highest risk of complications of influenza, such as transplant recipients	Pre-exposure	Duration of influenza activity
Unvaccinated people at high risk of complications of influenza in conjunction with vaccination when influenza activity is present in the community	Pre-exposure	14 days or until vaccine effectiveness is likely achieved
Unvaccinated people in close contact, including health care professionals, with people at high risk of influenza complications if unable to vaccinate, high-risk contacts cannot take chemoprophylaxis, and influenza is present in the community.	Pre-exposure	Duration of influenza activity

Patient Cases

Patient Case 6–1 SOAP Note

Collect	Chief complaint (CC)
Subjective	CR is a 26-year-old pregnant patient who presents to your pharmacy asking for a flu test. History of present illness (HPI) "I'm wondering if I would be able to get a flu test. I have a dry cough, sore throat, stuffy nose, fatigue, and body ache, which began last night. I'm not sure if it's the flu or a cold." Flu-like symptoms began <24 hours ago.

Objective	Medication list:
	• Prenatal vitamin daily
	• Acetaminophen as needed for fever and pain
	• Tri-Linyah (discontinued)
	Vaccination history:
	• Received all childhood vaccines
	• Tdap: 2023 with current pregnancy
	• COVID-19: Last booster (Moderna) December 2022
	• Flu: November 2022 (Fluarix Quadrivalent)
	Allergies: no known drug allergies (NKDA)
	Physical examination (PE)
	• Pregnant with first child, 2nd trimester
	• Vital signs
	  • Height: 66 in
	  • Weight: 145 lbs
	  • BMI: 23.4 kg/m^2
	  • BP: 136/82 mm HG
	  • Pulse: 72 beats/minute
	  • Respiratory rate: 60 breaths/minute
	  • Temperature: 101.5°F
	  • O$_2$ saturation: 98%
	Laboratory tests
	• Rapid influenza diagnostic test: positive influenza A, negative influenza B, Miscellaneous
	• Influenza in your area is currently high per the CDC Weekly U.S. Map: Influenza Summary Update, and patient lives close to the pharmacy.

Assess	Based on symptoms and symptom onset, CR is high risk for influenza. The result of RIDT is positive for influenza A, based on flu activity this is likely a true positive result. Pregnant women are at risk for influenza-related complications. Patient has no contraindications to antiviral therapy for influenza. Patient is up to date for vaccinations during pregnancy. Symptom onset was within 24 hours; medication is most effective when taken when symptomatic for no more than 48 hours.
Plan	Patient is a candidate for antiviral therapy as pregnant women are at risk for influenza-related complications. Oral oseltamivir is the preferred treatment for influenza during pregnancy. Baloxavir should be avoided during pregnancy; no human data is available. Zanamivir may be considered in pregnant patients but is less preferred compared to oseltamivir. Recommend: Oseltamivir 75 mg twice daily for 5 days. Goal is to reduce duration of influenza symptoms and reduce severity of illness.

Patient Case 6–1 SOAP Note cont'd

Implement	Prescribe oseltamivir 75 mg twice daily for 5 days based on state protocol. Notify patient's OB-GYN and PCP that oseltamivir has been prescribed. Counsel patient that medication should be taken as soon as possible, as it is most effective when taken within 36–48 hours of symptom onset. Counsel patient about potential adverse effects, including nausea, vomiting, and allergic reactions such as rash and facial swelling.
Monitor/ Follow-up	Schedule follow-up call with patient after 5 days to ensure patient took medication as prescribed. If symptoms persist or worsen after 5 days, refer patient to PCP.

Patient Case 6–2 SOAP Note

Collect	CC
Subjective	JW is a 75-year-old man who presents to the pharmacy requesting a flu test. HPI "I haven't been feeling well the past few days, and I want to see if I have the flu." Flu-like symptoms began "about 2 to 3 days ago." Symptoms include body ache, cough, fatigue, fever, chest congestion, shortness of breath, nausea, and sneezing.

Objective	Past medical history (PMH):
	• Diabetes
	• Hypertension
	• COPD
	Social history (SH): ex-smoker (20 pack year history)
	Medication list:
	• Metformin 1000 mg twice daily
	• Lisinopril 20 mg daily
	• Atorvastatin 40 mg daily
	• Advair Diskus 500 mcg/100 mcg twice daily
	• ASA 81 mg daily
	• Albuterol HFA inhaler as needed
	Vaccination history:
	• Tdap: 2020
	• Pneumovax 23: 2013
	• COVID-19: last booster (Comirnaty) December 2022
	• Flu: October 2022 (Fluzone HD Quadrivalent)
	Allergies: NKDA
	PE
	• Vital signs
	  • Height: 71 in
	  • Weight: 245 lbs
	  • BMI: 34.2 kg/m2
	  • BP: 138/88 mm HG
	  • Pulse: 80 beats/minute
	  • Respiratory rate: 70 breaths/minute
	  • Temperature: 100.8°F
	  • O2 saturation: 94%
	Laboratory tests
	• Rapid influenza diagnostic test: negative influenza A, negative influenza B
	• A1C: 7.1%
	• Total cholesterol (TC): 202 mg/dL; HDL: 40 mg/dL, LDL: 100 mg/dL
	Misc: Influenza in your area is currently high per the CDC Weekly U.S. Map: Influenza Summary Update, and patient lives close to the pharmacy.

Patient Case 6–2 SOAP Note cont'd

Assess	Based on symptoms and symptom onset, JW is at high risk for influenza. The result of RIDT is negative for influenza A and B. Based on flu activity, type of test, and time between onset of symptoms and testing, there is potential for a false negative result. Patient is over the age of 65 and has other conditions (COPD and diabetes) that place him at high risk of influenza-related complications. Decreased oxygen saturation and shortness of breath may be indicative of severe influenza, pneumonia, or exacerbation of COPD. Patient is at increased risk for pneumonia as he is not up to date with pneumococcal vaccination. Renal function labs are not currently available, but patient may have decreased renal function based on age and other medical conditions.
Plan	Influenza test results should be confirmed with a molecular assay. Patient is not up to date with pneumococcal vaccination, and concomitant conditions place him at a higher risk for pneumonia. Patient should be referred for molecular assay influenza test and assessment for pneumonia.
Implement	Refer patient to emergency department for molecular assay influenza test and assessment for pneumonia. A copy of the negative RIDT influenza test results may be provided to the patient and sent to the PCP to be included in his electronic health record. Patient may be empirically started on influenza antivirals upon admission to the hospital while awaiting test results.
Monitor/ Follow-up	Follow-up with patient or caregiver via telephone to ensure he sought medical care.

References

1. Centers for Disease Control and Prevention. Pinkbook: Influenza. Atlanta, GA: CDC. Available at: https://www.cdc.gov/vaccines/pubs/pinkbook/flu.html. Accessed March 30, 2023.

2. Centers for Disease Control and Prevention. Types of Influenza Viruses. Atlanta, GA: CDC. Available at: https://www.cdc.gov/flu/about/viruses/types.htm. Accessed March 30, 2023.

3. Centers for Disease Control and Prevention. Background and Epidemiology. Atlanta, GA: CDC. Available at: https://www.cdc.gov/flu/professionals/acip/background-epidemiology.htm. Accessed March 30, 2023.

4. Centers for Disease Control and Prevention. Burden of Influenza. Atlanta, GA: CDC. Available at: https://www.cdc.gov/flu/about/burden/index.html. Accessed March 30, 2023.

5. Centers for Disease Control and Prevention. New Study Identifies Racial and Ethnic Disparities in Severe Flu Outcomes. Atlanta, GA: CDC. Available at: https://www.cdc.gov/flu/spotlights/2020-2021/racial-ethnic-disparities-severe-flu-outcomes.htm. Accessed March 30, 2023.

6. Centers for Disease Control and Prevention. Flu Symptoms & Complications. Atlanta, GA: CDC. Published October 3, 2022. Accessed March 28, 2023. Available at: https://www.cdc.gov/flu/symptoms/symptoms.htm

7. Gaitonde DY, Moore FC, Morgan MK. Influenza: Diagnosis and treatment. *Am Fam Physician*. 2019;100(12):751–758.

8. Uyeki TM, Bernstein HH, Bradley JS, et al. Clinical Practice Guidelines by the Infectious Diseases Society of America: 2018 Update on Diagnosis, Treatment, Chemoprophylaxis, and Institutional Outbreak Management of Seasonal Influenza. *Clinical Infectious Diseases*. 2019;68(6):e1-e47. doi:10.1093/cid/ciy866

9. National Institutes of Health. Is It Flu, COVID-19, Allergies, or a Cold? Staying Healthy This Winter. Bethesda, MD: NIH. Available at: https://newsinhealth.nih.gov/2022/01/it-flu-covid-19-allergies-or-cold. Accessed January 23, 2024.

10. Centers for Disease Control and Prevention. Flu: What To Do If You Get Sick. Atlanta, GA: CDC. Available at: https://t.cdc.gov/2S48. Accessed April 3, 2023.

11. Centers for Disease Control and Prevention. Overview of Influenza Testing Methods. Atlanta, GA: CDC. Available at: https://www.cdc.gov/flu/professionals/diagnosis/overview-testing-methods.htm. Accessed March 30, 2023.

12. Centers for Disease Control and Prevention. Rapid Influenza Diagnostic Tests (RIDTs). Atlanta, GA: CDC. Available at: https://www.cdc.gov/flu/professionals/diagnosis/table-ridt.html. Accessed March 31, 2023.

13. Centers for Disease Control and Prevention. Nucleic Acid Detection Based Tests. Atlanta, GA: CDC. Available at: https://www.cdc.gov/flu/professionals/diagnosis/table-nucleic-acid-detection.html. Accessed March 31, 2023.

14. UpToDate Inc. Acetaminophen Oral. Drug Facts and Comparisons online, Facts and Comparisons eAnswers online. Waltham, MA: UpToDate. Available at: https://fco.factsandcomparisons.com. Accessed January 24, 2024.

15. UpToDate Inc. Ibuprofen Oral. Drug Facts and Comparisons online, Facts and Comparisons eAnswers online. Waltham, MA: UpToDate. Available at: https://fco.factsandcomparisons.com. Accessed January 24, 2024.

16. UpToDate Inc. Naproxen Oral. Drug Facts and Comparisons online, Facts and Comparisons eAnswers online. Waltham, MA: UpToDate. Available at: https://fco.factsandcomparisons.com. Accessed January 24, 2024.

17. National Center for Complementary and Integrative Health. Flu and Colds: In Depth. Bethesda, MD: NCCAM. Available at: https://www.nccih.nih.gov/health/flu-and-colds-in-depth. Accessed January 23, 2024.

18. Centers for Disease Control and Prevention. Influenza Antiviral Medications: Clinician Summary. Atlanta, GA: CDC. Available at: https://www.cdc.gov/flu/professionals/antivirals/summary-clinicians.htm. Accessed March 30, 2023.

19. National Alliance of State Pharmacy Associations. Pharmacist Prescribing: "Test and Treat." Richmond, VA: NASPA. Available at: https://naspa.us/resource/pharmacist-prescribing-for-strep-and-flu-test-and-treat/. Accessed April 3, 2023.

20. Hohmeier KC, McKeirnan K, Akers J, et al. Implementing community pharmacy-based influenza point-of-care test-and-treat under collaborative practice agreement. *Implement Sci Commun*. 2022 Jul 16;3(1):77. doi:10.1186/s43058-022-00324-z

21. Hardin R, Roberts P, Hudspeth B, et al. Development and Implementation of an Influenza Point-Of-Care Testing Service in a Chain Community Pharmacy Setting. *Pharmacy (Basel)*. 2020 Oct 6;8(4):182. doi:10.3390/pharmacy8040182

22. Centers for Disease Control and Prevention. Rapid Influenza Diagnostic Tests (RIDTs). Atlanta, GA: CDC. Available at: https://www.cdc.gov/flu/professionals/diagnosis/clinician_guidance_ridt.htm. Accessed January 24, 2024.

CHAPTER 7

Streptococcal Infection

Megan G. Smith, PharmD, BCACP

Key Points

- Noninvasive Group A streptococcal (GAS) infections are the most common types of infections in outpatient settings and include strep throat, scarlet fever, and impetigo.
- GAS infections are more prevalent among children aged 5–15 years old, and they are more common in the winter and spring seasons.
- GAS infections are self-limiting, but people who are appropriately treated with antibiotics become non-contagious after 24 hours of treatment.
- Patients who have a history of rheumatic fever, immunosuppression, or recurrent pharyngitis should be referred to a primary care provider (PCP) for further diagnostic evaluation.
- The modified Centor score is a clinical prediction tool that identifies patients who are at low risk for GAS and do not need further testing or treatment.
- The treatment of choice is penicillin or amoxicillin.

Group A streptococcal (GAS) disease is caused by the bacterium *Streptococcus pyogenes* and can result in either invasive or noninvasive infections. Invasive GAS infections are closely monitored by the Centers for Disease Control and Prevention (CDC) as they can lead to serious illnesses such as cellulitis or streptococcal toxic shock syndrome. CDC reported a prevalence of 20,270 cases and 1,870 deaths from invasive GAS disease in 2020.[1]

Noninvasive GAS infections, on the other hand, are the most common types of infections in outpatient settings and include pharyngitis (strep throat), scarlet fever, and impetigo. While these infections are not monitored yearly by CDC, the World Health Organization estimated 616 million new cases of strep pharyngitis each year in 2005.[2] A more recent meta-analysis found that the pooled incidence rate for sore throat was 82 episodes per 100 child years, while the pooled incidence rate for GAS was 22.1 episodes per 100 child years.[3]

GAS infections are more prevalent among children aged 5–15 years, and they are more common in the winter and spring seasons. The most common mode of transmission for GAS infections is through direct person-to-person contact via respiratory droplets.[4] Group A streptococcus causes 20%–30% of sore throats in children and 5%–15% of sore throats in adults. Generally, GAS infections are self-limiting, and symptoms can resolve on their own within a week or two without any specific treatment.[4] However, people who are appropriately treated with antibiotics become non-contagious after 24 hours of treatment. Therefore, it is essential to seek medical attention for patients with symptoms of a GAS infection, especially if at a higher risk, such as young children or those with weakened immune systems. Prompt diagnosis and treatment can prevent complications and reduce the spread of GAS infections.

Clinical Prevalence of Group A Streptococcus

When diagnosing a GAS infection in a patient, it is essential to differentiate between viral and bacterial infections (Table 7–1). Viral pharyngitis can be diagnosed through patient history and clinical examination, with symptoms including cough, rhinorrhea, hoarseness, and conjunctivitis.[4] On the other hand, Group A pharyngitis, which is caused by bacteria, presents with sudden-onset sore throat, pain when swallowing, and fever, often accompanied by inflammation of the pharynx and tonsils, patchy exudates, and swollen cervical lymph nodes. Other symptoms of bacterial infection can include malaise, headache, nausea, abdominal pain, and vomiting.[5]

Table 7–1. Comparison of viral and bacterial pharyngitis

Viral	Bacterial
Cough	Sudden-onset sore throat
Rhinorrhea	Fever
Hoarseness	Inflammation of tonsils with exudates
Conjunctivitis	Swollen cervical lymph nodes, malaise, headache

It is important to be aware of the potential complications that can arise from bacterial infections, particularly untreated Group A pharyngitis. Acute post-streptococcal glomerulonephritis (APSGN) and acute rheumatic fever (ARF) are two such complications.[5] ARF is a systemic disorder that can develop because of untreated GAS pharyngeal infection and can lead to arthritis, carditis, and neurological symptoms. The incidence of ARF is 8 to 51 per 100,000 people worldwide, and it most commonly affects children 5 to 15 years old following a GAS infection.[6] APSGN is a kidney disorder that occurs due to an immune complex-mediated response and can cause symptoms such as edema, hypertension, urinary sediment abnormalities, and decreased levels of complement components in the serum.[5] The estimated worldwide burden of APSGN is approximately 472,000 cases per year, with approximately 404,000 cases being reported in children and 456,000 cases occurring in less developed countries.[7]

Patients who have a history of rheumatic fever, immunosuppression, or recurrent pharyngitis should be referred to a PCP for further diagnostic evaluation. By recognizing the symptoms of both viral and bacterial infections and being aware of their potential complications, HCPs can make informed decisions regarding diagnosis, treatment, and management of patients.

Diagnosis

When diagnosing GAS pharyngitis, HCPs must use either a rapid antigen detection test (RADT) or throat culture if there are no clear viral symptoms.[8] RADTs have high specificity for GAS, but their sensitivity is more variable than that of the throat culture test, which is considered the gold standard diagnostic test. To diagnose GAS pharyngitis, the American Academy of Family Physicians, the Centers for Disease Control, and the American College of Physicians recommend using a clinical prediction model based on signs and symptoms in addition to the RADT.[8,9]

The strongest independent predictors of GAS pharyngitis are patient age between 5 and 15 years, absence of cough, tender anterior cervical adenopathy, tonsillar exudates, and fever.[10] To diagnose GAS pharyngitis, a RADT should be ordered in patients with a modified Centor score of 2 or more. The modified Centor score (Table 7–2) is a clinical prediction tool that identifies patients who are at low risk for GAS and do not need further testing or treatment.[11] The score is calculated based on the presence or absence of five clinical factors: fever, tonsillar exudates, swollen and tender lymph nodes, absence of cough, and age. Scores of 0 or 1 carry a low risk of GAS infection and do not require further testing or treatment, while scores of 2 or more require a RADT and/or throat culture to confirm the diagnosis.

A study of more than 200,000 patients validated the modified Centor score and showed that it more precisely classified the risk of GAS infection among patients with a sore throat.[12] Scores of 0 carried a risk of 8% for GAS, scores of 1 carried a risk of 14%, scores of 2 carried a risk of 23%, scores of 3 carried a risk of 37%, and scores of 4 or more carried a risk of 55%. Incorporating the modified Centor score into guidelines can help HCPs identify patients who are at low risk for GAS infection and do not need further testing or treatment while ensuring that patients with higher scores receive appropriate diagnosis and treatment.

Table 7-2. Modified Centor score assessment[9]

Age	☐ 3-14 years: +1 ☐ 15-44: 0 ☐ ≥ 45 years: -1
Exudate or swelling on tonsils	☐ No: 0 ☐ Yes: +1
Tender/swollen anterior cervical lymph nodes	☐ No: 0 ☐ Yes: +1
Temperature >100.4°F	☐ No: 0 ☐ Yes: +1
Cough	☐ Present: 0 ☐ Absent: +1

Physical Assessment

Thorough collection of vital signs, including blood pressure, respiratory rate, and oxygen saturation, is important to evaluate whether the patient is clinically stable. After determining that the patient is stable and further evaluation is appropriate, physical assessment techniques that may be used to identify components of the modified Centor score are as follows.[10]

Tonsillar exudates: Inspection of the oropharynx can help detect the presence of tonsillar exudates, which are white or yellow spots or patches on the tonsils (Figure 7-1). A light source and tongue depressor may be used to facilitate examination.

Figure 7-1. Tonsillar exudates and white patches on swollen tonsils

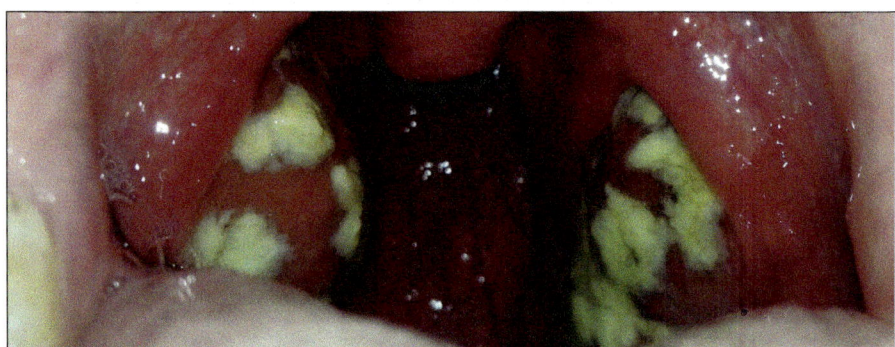

Tender anterior cervical lymphadenopathy or lymphadenitis: Palpation of the anterior cervical lymph nodes can detect tenderness, swelling, or lymphadenopathy, which are common signs of group A beta-hemolytic streptococci pharyngitis (GABHS). (Source: This image available in the creative commons license at: https://images.app.goo.gl/x6jAK2RFbEgMySPf9)

Absence of cough: Observing and asking the patient if they have experienced coughing or wheezing can help identify the absence of cough.

Temperature: Taking an oral or temporal temperature and asking the patient about their history of fever can help identify whether they meet the fever criteria for the modified Centor score.

Point-of-Care Testing

POCTs for GAS work by detecting the presence of bacterial antigens or DNA in a patient's throat swab sample. These tests use immunochromatographic or nucleic acid amplification technology (NAAT) to detect GAS antigens or DNA, respectively.[9,13-15] See Table 7-3 for select POCTs.

In immunochromatographic tests, a patient's throat swab is mixed with a reagent that contains antibodies that specifically recognize GAS antigens. If GAS is present in the sample, the antibodies will bind to the bacterial antigens, forming a visible line on the test strip. The presence of this line indicates a positive test result for GAS.

In NAAT, a patient's throat swab is mixed with a reagent that amplifies any GAS DNA present in the sample using polymerase chain reaction (PCR) technology. The amplified DNA is then detected using fluorescent probes or other detection methods. A positive test result for GAS indicates the presence of GAS DNA in the sample.

Both types of POCTs for GAS are relatively simple to perform and can provide results within minutes, allowing HCPs to diagnose GAS pharyngitis and prescribe appropriate treatment promptly. However, these tests are not always 100% accurate, and some patients may require additional confirmatory testing using a throat culture assay.

Table 7-3. Comparison of POCT devices for Group A Streptococcus

CLIA-waived test type	Example brands	Cost	Key points
Immunoassay, antigen, dipstick	Quidel QuickVue OSOM STREP A TEST	$	• All-in-one kit • Least amount of space and equipment needed • Usually lowest sensitivity of the 3 options • Results within 5 minutes
Immunoassay, antigen, instrument-based	Quidel Sofia 2[13] BD Veritor	$$	• Scan and "walk away" features • Options for memory storage, printouts, and connectivity to local trends • Option to test multiple samples simultaneously • Results within 5 minutes
Nucleic acid amplification by PCR	Roche Cobas Liat[14] Accula Strep A Test[15] Xpert Xpress Strep A test Alere i Strep A 2	$$$	• Barcode and touchscreen systems included • Local trend reporting • Usually highest sensitivity of the three options • Results within 20 minutes

Treatment of GAS

To diagnose GAS pharyngitis, the American Academy of Family Physicians, the Centers for Disease Control and Prevention, and the American College of Physicians recommend using a clinical prediction model based on signs and symptoms in addition to the RADT.[8,9] Figure 7-2 outlines the patient assessment, referral, and diagnosis of GAS pharyngitis.

Figure 7–2. Patient assessment and diagnosis algorithm for GAS pharyngitis

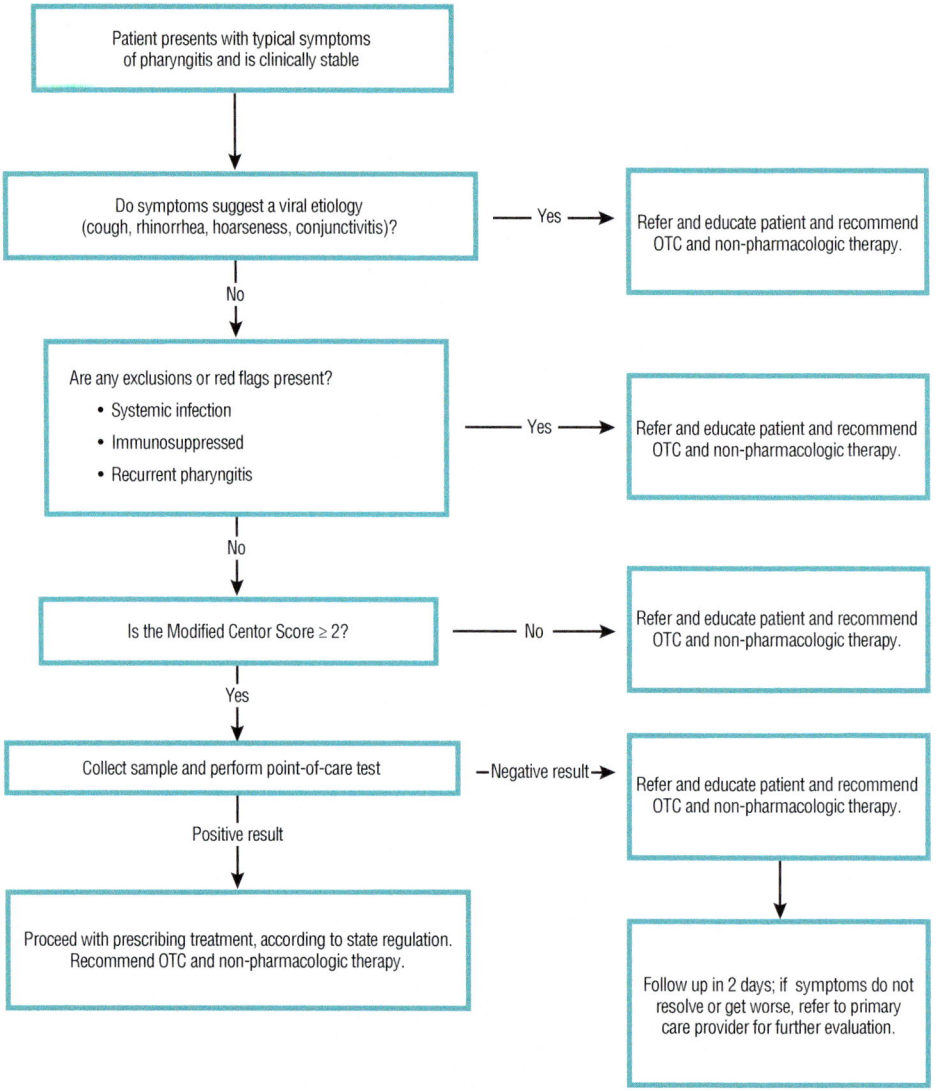

Treatment Recommendations

The treatment of GAS infection aims to relieve symptoms, prevent complications, and prevent the spread of the infection to others.[8] The most effective way to achieve these goals is through antibiotic therapy initiated within a few days of symptom onset. According to the 2012 guidelines from the Infectious Diseases Society of America (IDSA), GAS infection is uncommon in children younger than 3 years.[16] Therefore, diagnosis and treatment should be considered carefully in this age group.

All patients with pharyngitis, regardless of the cause, should be offered appropriate doses of analgesics and antipyretics, as well as other supportive care. These practices can help relieve symptoms and make the patient more comfortable while the infection is being treated. See Figure 7–3 for a summary of treatment recommendations, including nonpharmacologic therapy and supportive care.

Antipyretic and analgesic OTC options include[17]:

- Adults
    - Acetaminophen 650 mg every 4 to 6 hours as needed (maximum daily dose: 4000 mg)
    - Ibuprofen 200 mg every 4 to 6 hours as needed for 10 days for pain or for 3 days for fever (maximum daily dose: 1200 mg)
- Pediatrics
    - Acetaminophen 10 to 15 mg/kg/dose every 4 to 6 hours as needed (maximum daily dose: 75 mg/kg)
    - Ibuprofen 5 to 10 mg/kg/dose (maximum dose: 600 mg/dose) every 6 to 8 hours (maximum daily dose: 40 mg/kg)

GAS remains universally sensitive and has no known resistance to penicillin, making it the drug of choice for treating GAS infections.[9] Antibiotics such as cephalosporins and macrolides are also used clinically as alternatives or in cases of penicillin allergy. According to the IDSA guidelines, a 10-day treatment course with either penicillin or amoxicillin is recommended for the management of GABHS infection.[16] These antibiotics are cost-effective, have a narrow-spectrum, and are associated with low incidences of adverse effects. For individuals who are allergic to these antibiotics, the IDSA suggests prescribing first-generation cephalosporin for 10 days or azithromycin for 5 days.

Studies have shown that antibiotic therapy initiated within a few days of symptom onset can decrease the duration of symptoms by 1 to 2 days.[11] It is important to follow the full course of antibiotics as prescribed, even if symptoms improve before the medication is finished, to ensure that the infection is fully treated and to prevent the development of antibiotic-resistant bacteria.

Figure 7–3. Treatment recommendations for GAS pharyngitis

Non-pharmacological

- Lozenges or drops containing menthol, dyclonine, benzocaine, or hexylresorcinol
- Throat spray containing phenol or benzocaine
- Cold food provides hydration and numbing. Soft foods preferable.
- Tea or honey coats throat to help relieve pain and irritation

Self-Care

- Acetaminophen (dose in text)
- Ibuprofen (dose in text)

1st Line Treatment

- Amoxicillin
    - Adults: 500 mg twice daily or 1 g once daily for 10 days
    - Pediatrics: 50 mg/kg/day once daily or in divided doses every 12 hours for 10 days
- Penicillin V
    - Adults: 500 mg 2 to 3 times daily for 10 days
    - Children ≤27 kg: Oral: 250 mg every 8 to 12 hours for 10 days
    - Children >27 kg and Adolescents: Oral: 500 mg every 8 to 12 for 10 days

2nd Line or Penicillin Allergy Alternative

- Cephalexin
    - Adults: 500 mg twice daily for 10 days
    - Pediatrics: 40 mg/kg/day divided every 12 hours for 10 days

3rd Line Treatment

- Azithromycin
    - Adults: 12 mg/kg (maximum: 500 mg) once daily for 5 days
    - Pediatrics: 12 mg/kg/dadose once daily for 5 days; maximum dose: 500 mg

Prescribing treatment may require a CPA or required use of state-approved protocols. Scope of practice and criteria will vary by state and pharmacists should contact their state board of pharmacy for current state-specific information. A summary is provided in Table 7–3.[18]

Table 7–3. Mechanism to prescribe for Strep POCT[16]

Direct prescribing authority	Colorado, Idaho
Direct prescribing authority using a statewide protocol	Arkansas, Delaware, Iowa, Kansas
Delegated prescribing authority/collaborative practice agreements	Florida, Idaho, Illinois, Kentucky, Michigan, Minnesota, Montana, Nebraska, New Mexico, North Dakota, South Dakota, Tennessee, Texas, Utah, Vermont, Washington, Wisconsin

Indications for Referral

Referral to a PCP or specialist may be necessary in cases of recurrent infections, complications, non-resolving symptoms, or signs and symptoms indicating a more serious infection or complication.[5]

If a patient has recurrent strep throat infections (more than 4 or 5 in a year), referral is necessary and may require a tonsillectomy to prevent future infections. Complications such as rheumatic fever, glomerulonephritis, and peritonsillar abscess require specialized treatment and management. If a patient's symptoms do not improve with antibiotics or return after treatment, the patient should be referred for alternative testing and evaluation. Finally, symptoms that indicate a more serious infection such as difficulty breathing, difficulty swallowing, severe throat pain, severe headache, high fever, and neck stiffness should also be referred.[5]

Patient Cases

Patient Case 7–1 SOAP Note

Collect	Chief Complaint
Subjective	A 47-year-old woman presents to the pharmacy with a sore throat.
	HPI
	"I have a sore throat and think I may have strep."
	Started yesterday
	Past medical history (PMH): diabetes, never had strep throat before
	The patient presents with sore throat that started yesterday and is wondering if she has strep. To her knowledge, she has not been around anyone else with an infection.
Objective	Medication list: metformin and Byetta
	Allergies: no known drug allergies (NKDA)
	Review of symptoms (ROS): sore throat with cough, some chills and fatigue
	General appearance: appropriately groomed, no signs of distress, has large scarf wrapped around shoulders
	Physical examination (PE): cough noted and clear nasal discharge consistent with rhinorrhea
	Vital signs (VS):
	BP: 128/92 mm HG
	Respiratory rate: 14 breaths/minute
	O2 saturation: 98%
	Temperature: 101.2°F
	Head, ears, eyes, nose, and throat examination (HEENT):
	Neck/lymph nodes: absence of tender or swollen anterior cervical lymph nodes
	Lungs/thorax (or chest): negative for exudate or swelling on the tonsils
Assess	The patient is clinically stable. Based on the subjective and objective information, sore throat and fever are consistent with GAS pharyngitis, but the modified Centor score is 0: presence of cough (0), absence of swollen tonsils and lymph nodes (0), temperature (+1), age (–1). Therefore, the likelihood of a GAS infection is very low. The presence of cough and nasal discharge are indicative of a viral infection.
Plan	The goal is to relieve pain, reduce fever, and reduce the spread of the virus. Supportive measures such as non-pharmacological and over-the-counter antipyretics are the best choices.
	Referral to PCP if symptoms do not improve in the next 1–2 days or the patient shows signs of a complication or serious infections such as stiff neck, severe headache, or difficulty swallowing or breathing.
	Patient can still elect to be tested for GAS if cost is not a barrier.
Implement	Educate the patient on the assessment of viral versus bacterial infection and to avoid close contact with others until 24 hours after fever has resolved.
	Recommend acetaminophen 650 mg by mouth every 6 hours for the next two days, then as needed for pain management. Recommend lozenges with menthol and hot tea to reduce irritation in the throat.
Monitor/ Follow-Up	Follow-up with patient in two days to assess response and resolution of symptoms. Viral infections are self-limiting within 2 weeks. If symptoms have not resolved or are worsening, coordinate referral to PCP.

Patient Case 7-2 SOAP Note

Collect	Chief Complaint
Subjective	A 15-year-old boy and his mother present to the pharmacy with a sore throat. "My throat hurts and it is hard to swallow."
	HPI
	Started two days ago
	PMH: no history of strep throat, negative for any respiratory infections in the last month
	The patient presents with sore throat that started two days ago and a couple of his classmates have just been diagnosed with strep throat.
Objective	Medication list: none
	Allergies: NKDA
	ROS: Sore throat, some fatigue
	General appearance: well-nourished, febrile, appears tired but no signs of distress
	PE: skin is cool and pale
	VS:
	BP: 134/96 mm Hg
	RR: 14 breaths/minute
	O2 saturation: 97%
	Temperature: 101.0°F
	Height: 55 in
	Weight: 95 lb
	Head, ears, eyes, nose, and throat examination (HEENT):
	Neck/lymph nodes: absence of tender or swollen anterior cervical lymph nodes
	Lungs/thorax (or chest): tonsils are red, swollen and have small white patches
	RADT result for group A streptococcus: positive
Assess	The patient is clinically stable. Based on the subjective and objective information, signs and symptoms are consistent with GAS pharyngitis. The modified Centor score is 3: absence of cough (+1), presence of swelling and exudate on tonsils (+1), temperature (+1), and age (0). Therefore, the likelihood of a GAS infection is high and it is appropriate to perform a POCT. The test result is positive, confirming the diagnosis of GAS pharyngitis.
Plan	The goal is to eradicate infection, relieve pain, reduce fever, and reduce the spread of the virus. Antibiotic therapy is indicated, and the infection is most sensitive to penicillin. Recommend amoxicillin 1000 mg once daily for 10 days.
	Supportive measures such as non-pharmacological and over-the-counter antipyretics are recommended to provide comfort while treating the infection.
Implement	Educate the patient on the use and adverse effects of amoxicillin and to finish the full course regardless of whether symptoms are improving. Avoid close contact with others until 24 hours after the fever has resolved and the patient has started taking the antibiotic. Practice good hand hygiene and cover any coughs or sneezes to help reduce the spread of infection to others.
	Recommend acetaminophen 650 mg by mouth every 6 hours for the next two days, then as needed for pain management. Recommend lozenges with menthol and hot tea to reduce irritation in the throat.
Monitor/ Follow-Up	Follow-up with PCP if temperature increases or symptoms worsen. Recommend to the HCP to follow-up in 5 days to assess the patient's response and resolution of symptoms. Encourage the patient to finish the full ten days of treatment.

References

1. Centers for Disease Control and Prevention. CDC surveillance report 2020. Atlanta, GA: CDC. Available at: https://www.cdc.gov/abcs/downloads/GAS_Surveillance_Report_2020.pdf. Accessed March 31, 2023.

2. World Health Organization. *The Current Evidence for the Burden of Group A Streptococcal Diseases*. Geneva, Switzerland: WHO. Available at: https://apps.who.int/iris/handle/10665/69063. Accessed March 31, 2023.

3. Miller KM, Carapetis JR, Van Beneden CA, et al. The global burden of sore throat and group A *Streptococcus* pharyngitis: A systematic review and meta-analysis. *EClinicalMedicine*. 2022;20(48):101458. doi:10.1016/j.eclinm.2022.101458

4. Centers for Disease Control and Prevention. Group A Streptococcal (GAS) Disease. Atlanta, GA: CDC. Available at: https://www.cdc.gov/groupastrep/diseases-hcp/strep-throat.html. Accessed March 31, 2023.

5. Walker MJ, Barnett TC, McArthur JD, et al. Disease manifestations and pathogenic mechanisms of group A Streptococcus. *Clin Microbiol Rev*. 2014;27(2):264e301.

6. Lahiri S, Sanyahumbi A. Acute rheumatic fever. *Pediatr Rev*. 2021 May;42(5):221–232. doi:10.1542/pir.2019-0288

7. Ilyas M, Tolaymat A. Changing epidemiology of acute post-streptococcal glomerulonephritis in Northeast Florida: A comparative study. *Pediatric Nephrology*. 2008;23(7):1101–1106.

8. Cooper RJ, Hoffman JR, Bartlett JG, et al., for the American Academy of Family Physicians, American College of Physicians, American Society of Internal Medicine, Centers for Disease Control and Prevention. Principles of appropriate antibiotic use for acute pharyngitis in adults: Background. *Ann Intern Med*. 2001;134(6):509–517

9. Mustafa Z, Ghaffari M. Diagnostic Methods, Clinical Guidelines, and Antibiotic Treatment for Group A Streptococcal Pharyngitis: A Narrative Review. *Front Cell Infect Microbiol*. 2020 Oct 15;10:563627.

10. Kalra MG, Higgins KE, Perez ED. Common questions about Streptococcal Pharyngitis. *Am Fam Physician*. 2016 Jul 1;94(1):24–31. Erratum in: *Am Fam Physician*. 2017 Apr 1;95(7):414.

11. McIsaac WJ, White D, Tannenbaum D, Low DE. A clinical score to reduce unnecessary antibiotic use in patients with sore throat. *CMAJ*. 1998 Jan 13;158(1):75–83.

12. Fine AM, Nizet V, Mandl KD. Large-scale validation of the Centor and McIsaac scores to predict group A streptococcal pharyngitis. *Arch Intern Med*. 2012;172(11):847–852.

13. U.S. Food and Drug Administration. Sofia Strep A+ FIA. U.S. Food and Drug Administration Summary Letter. Silver Spring, MD: FDA. Available at: https://www.accessdata.fda.gov/cdrh_docs/pdf17/K171976.pdf. Accessed March 31, 2023.

14. U.S. Food and Drug Administration. Roche Liat Strep A Assay. U.S. Food and Drug Administration Summary Letter. Silver Spring, MD: FDA. Available at: https://www.accessdata.fda.gov/cdrh_docs/pdf14/K141338.pdf. Accessed March 31, 2023.

15. U.S. Food and Drug Administration. Accula Strep A Test. U.S. Food and Drug Administration Summary Letter. Silver Spring, MD: FDA. Available at: https://www.accessdata.fda.gov/cdrh_docs/pdf20/K201269.pdf. Accessed March 31, 2023.

16. Shulman ST, Bisno AL, Clegg HW, et al. Clinical practice guideline for the diagnosis and management of group A streptococcal pharyngitis: 2012 update by the Infectious Diseases Society of America. *Clin Infect Dis*. 2012;55(10):e86–e102.

17. U.S. Food and Drug Administration. Over-the-Counter (OTC) Monograph M013: Internal Analgesic, Antipyretic, and Antirheumatic Drug Products for Over-the-Counter Human Use. Silver Spring, MD: FDA. Available at: https://dps-admin.fda.gov/omuf/sites/omuf/files/monograph-documents/2022-10/OTC%20Monograph_M013-Internal%20Analgesic%2C%20Antipyretic%2C%20and%20Antirheumatic%20Drug%20Products%20for%20OTC%20Human%20Use%2010.14.2022.pdf. Accessed March 31, 2023.

18. National Alliance of State Pharmacy Associations. Pharmacist Prescribing: Test and Treat. Richmond, VA: NASPA. Available at: https://naspa.us/resource/pharmacist-prescribing-for-strep-and-flu-test-and-treat/. Accessed March 31, 2023.

CHAPTER 8

COVID-19 Testing

Traci M. Poole, PharmD, BCACP, BCGP

Key Points

- Information regarding the detection and treatment of COVID-19 is rapidly evolving. Pharmacists should aim to stay informed regarding current recommendations.
- Thorough assessment of the exposure and onset of symptoms is vital to the accuracy of POCT.
- Testing should be performed for anyone who presents with new-onset fever or upper respiratory symptoms.
- Pharmacists may continue to prescribe treatments to patients experiencing mild-to-moderate illness with risk factors for severe illness.

Severe acute respiratory syndrome coronavirus 2 (SARS-CoV-2) was identified as a novel pathogen that causes coronavirus disease 2019 (COVID-19) in early December 2019.[1] COVID-19 is extremely contagious and approximately 6.8 million deaths worldwide have been attributed to it.[2] It has devastated communities, crippled health care systems, and decimated economies.

Since the beginning of the pandemic, pharmacists in all settings have played and continue to play a key role in the prevention, diagnosis, and treatment of COVID-19. Community pharmacists are positioned to fill direct patient care needs, including dissemination of education, administration of vaccines, screening for illness, and appropriately recommending treatment for active infection.[3]

Important Terms

- Antigen—a toxin or other foreign substance that induces an immune response in the body, especially the production of antibodies.
- Antibody—a blood protein produced in response to and counteracting a specific antigen.
- Close contact—someone who was within 6 feet of an infected person for a total of 15 minutes or more in a 24-hour period.
- Nucleic Acid Amplification Test (NAAT)—a type of diagnostic test that uses a technique to amplify and detect genetic material of a virus or bacteria. These tests can include polymerase chain reaction (PCR), loop-mediated isothermal amplification (LAMP), and nucleic acid sequence-based amplification (NASBA).
- Sensitivity or Percent Positive Agreement (PPA)—a test's ability to designate an individual with infection as positive.
- Specificity or Negative Percent Agreement (NPA)—a test's ability to designate an individual who does not have an infection as negative.

SARS-CoV-2 is a member of the coronavirus family of viruses. The virus is spherical in shape with hallmark spike-like proteins on its surface. It binds to ACE2 receptors located in the heart, lungs, kidneys, and intestines to penetrate host cells for replication. Since the beginning of the pandemic, the virus has undergone several mutations, all of which have had their own unique characteristics with respect to contagiousness, clinical presentation, and severity of illness.[4]

At the time of writing, the current reported deaths in the United States as a result of COVID-19 infection are estimated at more than 1.1 million, but assumptions of attributable illness and death may be vastly underestimated.[5-7] As of 2024, the U.S. has experienced the highest number of infections and COVID-19–related deaths of any nation.[7] The cost burden of COVID-19 is not limited to the period of acute illness and extends for up to 6 months beyond diagnosis due to the lasting effects of infection, known as long COVID.[8] In 2020, it was reported by the Kaiser Family Foundation that one hospitalization for COVID-19 cost the health care system nearly $42,000.[9] Estimates purport that the overall cost of COVID-19 worldwide is between 10 and 22 trillion dollars.[10]

As of 2024, the incidence of cases worldwide is 437 million confirmed cases.[2] The local incidence of COVID-19 is based on several factors, including population density, social distancing, masking and testing policies, and vaccination rates. SARS-CoV-2 has undergone several mutations and reinfection is possible, but more time will be necessary to predict the behavior of the virus and its year-over-year prevalence and incidence as it continues to mutate and become endemic.

Person-to-person respiratory secretions have been identified as the primary means of SARS-CoV-2 transmission. Secondary means of SARS-CoV-2 transmission include infected surfaces; viral specimens have been identified in blood, stool, semen and ocular secretions, but the role of these modes of transmission in the spread of the virus is unclear. The average incubation period of SARS-CoV-2 is 5 to 6 days, with a range of up to 19 days.[11] Clinical disease progression usually occurs around day five with the initial presentation of symptoms. Worsening illness generally presents on day eight and will progress to critical illness within 16 days.[12]

While anyone may contract COVID-19, certain groups are associated with more exposure to the disease, including health care and essential business workers and those living in crowded or communal environments. Patients at risk for experiencing more severe illness include those who are unvaccinated, have certain underlying medical conditions (e.g., obesity, asthma, heart disease, diabetes, immunocompromised status), or age greater than 50 years, with risk markedly worsening after age 65.[13] After adjustment for age, studies have shown differences in the SARS-CoV-2 infection rate and illness severity among minority populations, which may reflect the consequences of increased exposure related to working in essential jobs, differences in living or transportation situations, lack of access to health care resources, and lower vaccination rates.[14,15]

Clinical Presentation of COVID-19

Clinical presentation of COVID-19 can vary from person to person, ranging from no symptoms to severe distress. Most patients in the outpatient setting are likely to experience mild-to-moderate illness and present commonly with fever, fatigue, myalgias, congestion, and cough. Other reported manifestations that may accompany those typical of upper respiratory illness include diarrhea, nausea, vomiting, and sudden loss of taste or smell. Complications of worsening illness include secondary infections such as pneumonia, blood clots, multisystem organ failure, and post–COVID-19 syndromes.[16]

Diagnosis

Early diagnosis is vital to reduce the transmission of COVID-19.[14] Due to the wide prevalence of COVID-19, the threshold for clinical suspicion of COVID-19 should be low. The possibility of a COVID-19 diagnosis should be considered in any patient presenting with upper respiratory illness symptoms or other commonly identified clinical manifestations of COVID-19. Due to the overlap of symptoms with other upper respiratory illnesses, patients will likely need to rule out influenza when presenting with these symptoms in the absence of known COVID-19 exposure.[17]

Physical assessment of patients presenting with symptoms of COVID-19 should include standard vitals and blood pressure to assess hemodynamic stability, collection of past medical history, weight and BMI to establish risk for severe illness, and an assessment of kidney and liver function through previous tests and diagnoses to determine eligibility for treatment if positive.

Available Tests

The optimal choice of test can vary based on the needs of the patient, such as screening or diagnostic testing. Various factors may influence the type of test chosen, including the required turnaround time for results, cost, and clinical presentation.

The gold standard for identification of COVID-19 remains laboratory-based moderate or high complexity NAATs, which detect viral ribonucleic acid (RNA) via various technologies such as PCR, LAMP, and NASPA. NAATs are highly sensitive and specific for SARS-CoV-2. While these tests take longer to obtain results in comparison with other tests (1–3 days), they are considered confirmatory for diagnosis. Pharmacists may be involved in collecting samples for these tests, but they are not able to perform them as they are not CLIA-waived. However, a small number of CLIA-waived rapid RT-PCR tests are available, which allow for administration at a pharmacy and produce results within 15–30 minutes. Rapid NAATs allow for earlier identification of infection with SARS-CoV-2, but these tests should not be used for serial testing for patients who have tested positive within the last 90 days.[18]

Rapid antigen tests are typically immunoassays designed to detect the nucleocapsid protein of SARS-CoV-2 antigens. These tests are up to 40% less sensitive than NAATs, which may result in an increased tendency to produce false negative results, but they are nearly as specific and are dependent on the viral load of an infected patient. Rapid antigen tests are ideal for patients presenting with symptoms and are best used when symptoms have been present for 48–96 hours. They typically produce results within 15 minutes or less and are more cost-effective than NAATs. The reduced sensitivity of rapid antigen tests in comparison with NAATs allows them to be used to preclude residual infection and permit patients to be released from quarantine.[20]

Antibody tests are serologic tests that utilize immunoassays to detect nucleocapsid or spike protein antibodies. Several CLIA-waived antibody tests are available. Antibody tests can be used to test for previous infection or the presence of antibodies after vaccination. However, the limited specificity and sensitivity of may lead to misinterpretation of a positive test since antibodies can be present both after infection and vaccination.[21] Antibody tests should not be used to identify active infection of COVID-19 or determine whether patients may leave quarantine or isolation.

Currently, all POCTs produce qualitative results, but many systems include diagnostic technology to limit user error and ensure accurate reading of results. Testing for COVID-19 also requires patient education to ensure that accurate results are obtained. For antigen tests, testing should occur around 48 hours after the onset of symptoms.[19] If a patient has been exposed to COVID-19, but remains asymptomatic, the patient should be encouraged to test for the virus on day five after the initial exposure. Since PCR tests are more sensitive than other types of tests, patients may use PCR tests as soon as symptoms appear. However, the 48-hour waiting period before testing should be applied for asymptomatic patients after exposure occurs.[22] Figure 8–1 provides an algorithmic approach to testing.

It is very important to understand the directions and limitations of each testing device. Each test may have unique characteristics regarding obtaining the sample, running the rest, or reading the results. It is advisable to provide testing services with all three types of tests to ensure that all surveillance and clinical needs of individual patients are met. Table 8–1 provides useful information for some of the most used tests.

Figure 8–1. COVID-19 testing algorithm

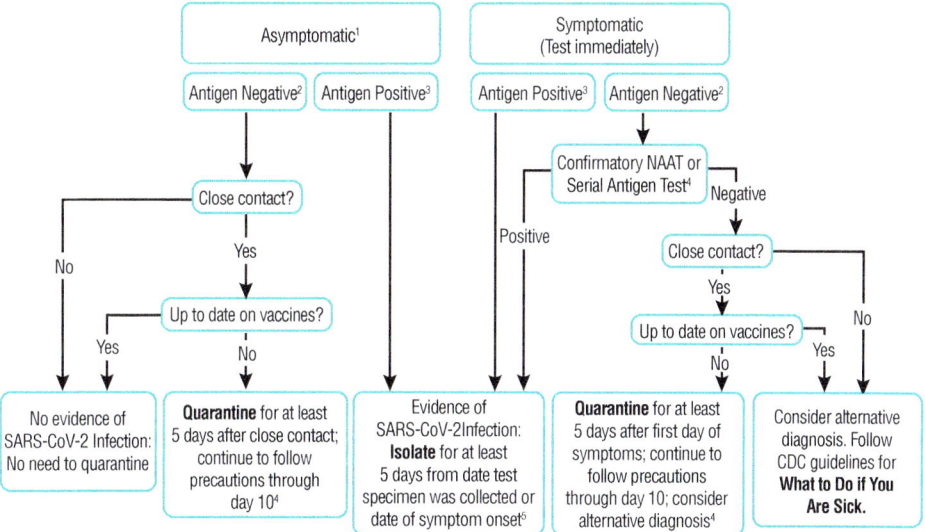

Source: Centers for Disease Control and Prevention.

1. If testing after a suspected exposure, test 5 days after last close contact with a person with COVID-19. For those who are traveling or have recently traveled, please refer to CDC's guidance for domestic and international travel during the COVID-19 pandemic. Take precautions while traveling.

2. Consider confirmatory testing with a NAAT or serial antigen testing for a negative antigen test result if the person has a higher likelihood of SARS-CoV-2 infection (e.g., in an area where the COVID-19 Community Level is high or the person has had close contact with or suspected exposure to someone infected with SARS-CoV-2) or if the person has symptoms of COVID-19.

3. A positive antigen test result generally does not require confirmatory testing; however, it could be considered when the person has a lower likelihood of infection (e.g., in an area where the COVID-19 Community Level is low and no known close contact with someone infected with SARS-CoV-2).

4. Confirmatory NAAT testing should take place as soon as possible after the antigen test, and not longer than 48 hours after the initial antigen testing. If the results are discordant, the confirmatory test result should be interpreted as definitive for the purposes of clinical diagnosis. If performing serial antigen testing, wait 24-48 hours between tests. See CDC's guidance on Quarantine and Isolation.

5. See CDC's guidance on treatments for COVID-19, particularly if individual is at high-risk of severe disease from COVID-19. Also see CDC's guidance on Quarantine and Isolation.

Table 8-1. Sample of available CLIA-waived COVID-19 point-of-care tests

Test	Type	PPA (sensitivity)	NPA (specificity)	Cost	Testing timeframe from symptom onset	Specimen
LumiraDx	Antigen	97.6%	96.6%	$$	12 days	Anterior nasal or nasopharyngeal
BD Veritor	Antigen	84%	100%	$$	5 days	Anterior nasal
Quidel Sofia	Antigen	96.7%	100%	$$	5 days	Anterior nasal
CareStart	Antigen	87.2% 93.8% (NP)	100% 99.3% (NP)	$	5 days	Anterior nasal or nasopharyngeal
Abbott ID Now	NAAT (RT-PCR)	94.7%	98.6%	$$$	7 days	Anterior nasal, nasopharyngeal, throat
Lucira	NAAT (RT-LAMP)	97%	98%	$$	n/a	Anterior nasal
Cepheid Xpert Xpress	NAAT (RT-PCR)	97.8%	95.6%	$$$$	n/a	Nasopharyngeal swab, nasal swab or nasal wash

Key: PPA, positive percent agreement; NPA, negative percent agreement; NP, nasopharyngeal.

Treatment

In September 2021, the U.S. Department of Health and Human Services updated the Public Readiness Emergency Preparedness Act (PREP Act) to allow pharmacists to identify patients who may benefit from early treatment with evidence of a positive test. It is unknown if this practice will continue after the PREP Act expires, but pharmacists with test-to-treat collaborative practice agreements or protocols may retain the ability to prescribe treatment for at-risk patients.[24]

Once a diagnosis of COVID-19 has been made, goals of therapy include reducing the severity of illness, prevention of hospitalization, shortening the duration of illness, and resolution of symptoms.[18] COVID-19 illness is treated based on the risk factors present for progression to severe illness and presentation of illness severity as defined in Table 8-2.[23]

The general treatment approach for COVID-19 encompasses both nonpharmacologic and pharmacologic treatment. Standard nonpharmacologic treatment should include adequate hydration, especially for those experiencing fever or other fluid losses from vomiting or diarrhea. Rest as needed is recommended; for those experiencing hypoxia, frequent repositioning and ambulation is necessary to maintain breathing capacity. Patients should be advised to return to activity as early as possible.[19]

Table 8-2. Classification of illness severity

Classification	Subjective findings	Objective findings
Asymptomatic	n/a	n/a
Mild	Fever, cough, sore throat, malaise/fatigue, headache, myalgia, N/V/D, anosmia, dysgeusia	Normal chest imaging
Moderate	Common clinical symptoms, but may include SOB	Radiologic evidence of lower respiratory tract infection; SpO2 ≥94% on room air
Severe	Common clinical symptoms plus marked tachypnea	SpO2 ≤94% on room air; PaO2/FiO2 <300; RR >30 breaths/min; lung infiltrates >50%

Adapted from Reference 21.

Evaluation of COVID-19 acuity is critical in outpatient settings. All patients are encouraged to utilize supportive symptomatic care as needed. Those with fever should utilize an antipyretic for fever and associated myalgias. Acetaminophen is preferred, but those who are unable to tolerate or fail treatment may utilize an NSAID such as ibuprofen. Cough suppressants are indicated if patients are experiencing disrupted sleep or significant discomfort. Other symptoms such as diarrhea may be treated using over-the-counter treatments as indicated.[19,23]

Treatment practices specific to COVID-19 are evolving and have undergone many iterations since the beginning of the pandemic. With each mutation of the original strain, some treatments have lost efficacy, requiring researchers and clinicians to pursue the development of viable treatment options for at-risk populations who are at increased risk for significant morbidity and mortality.[19,23]

Nirmatrelvir/ritonavir (Paxlovid; Pfizer Inc.) and remdesevir (Veklury; Gilead) are preferred first-line therapies for outpatient treatment of COVID-19, particularly in those at risk for severe illness. Pharmacy settings are generally not feasible locations for intravenous therapy with remdesevir, so referral is needed if it is the most viable treatment option. If patients are unable to access oral nirmatrelvir/ritonavir or remdesevir, or are clinically ineligible for treatment with these drugs, molnupiravir (Lagevrio; Merck) may be used as an alternative.[19]

Of note, it is required that prescribers have access to a current and full medication history, including renal and liver function test results, to safely prescribe these medications. Pharmacists must be prepared to manage complex drug interactions with the use of Paxlovid, but some pharmacists in community settings have found it difficult to quickly access interacting drug data from prescribers if they do not have access to electronic medical records. It is imperative to include solutions to this obstacle in the patient care process so that patients receive treatment in a timely manner. Figure 8-2 details which patients qualify for treatment other than supportive care.[19,23] At-home monitoring of SpO2 is recommended as a means of monitoring for worsening lung function and thus determining the need for further medical evaluation and treatment.

Figure 8–2. COVID-19 outpatient treatment algorithm

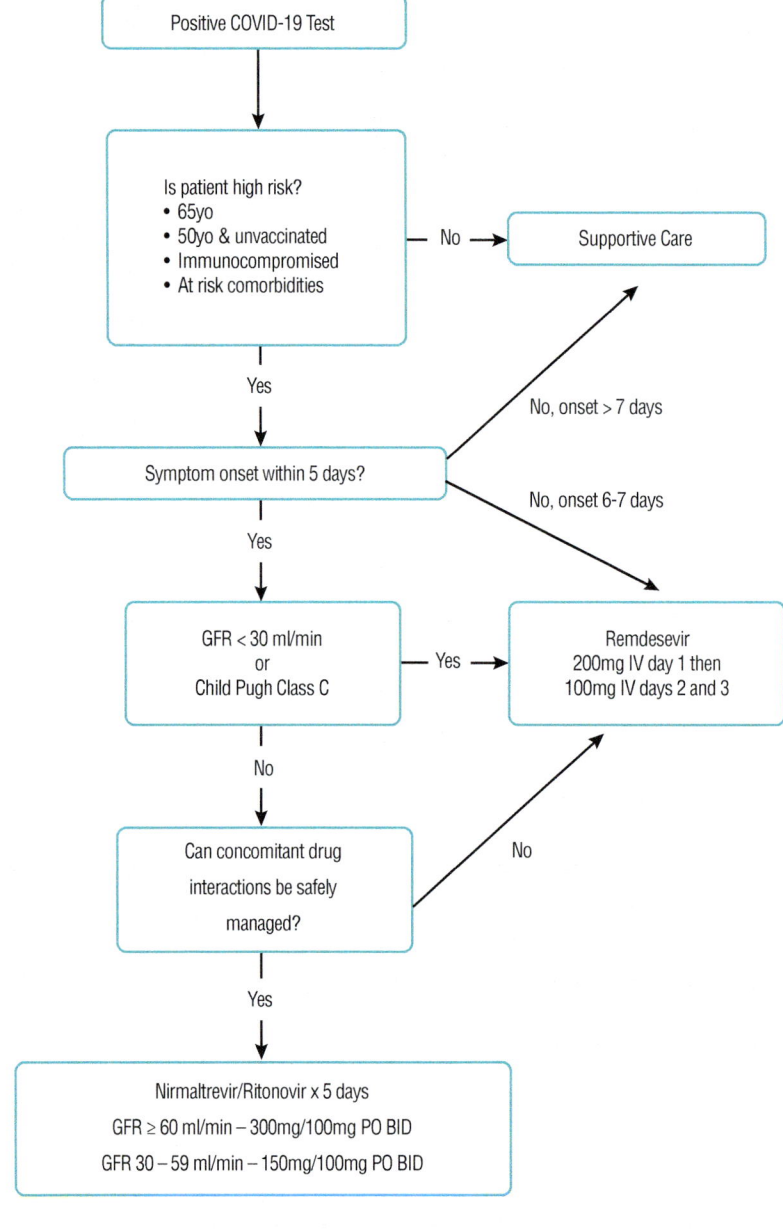

Patient Cases

Patient Case 8-1 SOAP Note

Collect **Subjective**	Chief complaint (CC)
	Patient presents to be tested for COVID-19
	History of present illness (HPI)
	52-year-old male complains of congestion, fatigue, headache, myalgia for 2 days. Patient was exposed 5 days ago to COVID-19
	Patient has received only the primary series of COVID-19 vaccinations
	Past medical history (PMH): obesity/hypertension (HTN)
Objective	Medication list: losartan/HCTZ 100/25 mg daily
	Allergies: no known drug allergies (NKDA)
	BP: 116/78 mm Hg; pulse: 78 bpm; respiratory rate (RR): 16 breaths/minute; temperature: 99.4°F; O2 saturation (SpO2): 98%; height: 72 in; weight: 232 lbs; glomerular filtration rate (GFR): 83 mL/min; no liver dysfunction
	COVID-19 rapid testing result: positive (+)
Assess	The patient presents with clear signs and symptoms of a mild viral upper respiratory illness. Based on his exposure and symptom timeline, he is an appropriate candidate for rapid antigen or rapid NAAT testing with a very small chance of a false positive result.
	Consider testing for both influenza A/B and COVID-19 if available to preclude dual infection or misdiagnosis in the absence of a positive COVID-19 test result.
	This patient is at risk for severe illness based on his past medical history. His comorbidities, symptom onset within 5 days, adequate liver and kidney function, and absence of relevant drug interactions qualify him for treatment with nirmatrelvir/ritonavir.
Plan	Counsel patient on nonpharmacologic measures such as adequate hydration, rest, appropriate level of tolerability to ambulate, and proper nutrition.
	Due to his mild clinical presentation and comorbidity of HTN, patient should be cautious when self-treating his symptoms with NSAIDs or pseudoephedrine products to avoid increases in his blood pressure.
	Recommend using acetaminophen for myalgias to avoid NSAID-induced elevation of blood pressure. May educate patient that if safer treatment modalities are not working, he could sparingly use less safe alternatives with regular blood pressure monitoring and discontinuation of NSAIDs or pseudoephedrine products if his blood pressure rises beyond his goal.
	Recommend: nirmatrelvir 300 mg 2 tablets by mouth twice daily ritonavir 100 mg 1 tablet by mouth twice daily
Implement	Encourage adherence to nirmatrelvir/ritonavir dosing regimen and vaccination with the bivalent COVID-19 booster as soon as he recovers from the present illness.
Monitor/ Follow-up	Patient should monitor RR and SpO2 and seek medical care if SpO2 is <95% or breaths per minute exceeds 20.
	If patient chooses to use less safe alternatives for myalgias/congestion, he should monitor his blood pressure daily and discontinue medications that can contribute to increased blood pressure if it is above his goal.
	If the patient experiences an allergic reaction to nirmatrelvir/ritonavir, he should discontinue the medication and call his PCP.

Patient Case 8–2 SOAP Note

Collect	Chief complaint
Subjective	Patient presents to be tested for COVID-19
	HPI
	74-year-old female complains of fever, myalgia, and recent onset of shortness of breath. Her initial symptom onset was 5 days ago with the shortness of breath presenting on day 4.
	Is current on all COVID-19 vaccination recommendations.
Objective	PMH: diabetes, hypertension, hypothyroidism
	Medication list: amlodipine 10 mg daily, metformin 1000 mg twice daily, levothyroxine 100 mcg daily
	Allergies: NKDA
	BP: 144/84 mm Hg; pulse: 92 bpm; RR: 24 breaths/minute; temperature: 101°F; SpO2: 93%; height: 72 in; weight: 232 lbs; GFR and liver function unknown
	COVID-19 rapid testing result: positive (+)
Assess	The patient presents with clear distress and signs and symptoms of a respiratory illness.
	Based on her symptom timeline, she is an appropriate candidate for rapid antigen or rapid NAAT testing.
	Should consider testing for both influenza A/B and COVID-19 if available to preclude dual infection or misdiagnosis in the absence of a positive COVID-19 test result.
	This patient is at risk for severe illness based on her past medical history and age.
	Her current clinical presentation indicates moderate-severe illness.
Plan	Based on her severity of illness and recent worsening of symptoms, she should be referred to the emergency department to obtain a full assessment of her clinical status and appropriateness of treatment.
Implement	Encourage the patient to seek immediate medical attention at the emergency department.
Monitor/ Follow-up	Call the patient in 3 days to check in on her clinical status and follow-up with the transitions of care initiated by the pharmacist.

References

1. Harapan H, Itoh N, Yufika A, et al. Coronavirus disease 2019 (COVID-19): A literature review. *Journal of Infection and Public Health*. 2020;13(5):667–673. doi:10.1016/j.jiph.2020.03.019

2. Worldometer. Coronavirus cases. Available at: https://www.worldometers.info/coronavirus/. Accessed April 11, 2023.

3. Pantasri T. Expanded roles of community pharmacists in covid-19: A scoping literature review. *Journal of the American Pharmacists Association*. 2022;62(3):649–657. doi:10.1016/j.japh.2021.12.013

4. Shirbhate E, Pandey J, Patel VK, et al. Understanding the role of ACE-2 receptor in pathogenesis of COVID-19 disease: a potential approach for therapeutic intervention. *Pharmacol Rep*. 2021;73(6):1539–1550. doi:10.1007/s43440-021-00303-6

5. Havers FP, Reed C, Lim T, et al. Seroprevalence of antibodies to SARS-CoV-2 in 10 sites in the United States, March 23–May 12, 2020. *JAMA Intern Med*. 2020;180(12):1576–1586. doi:10.1001/jamainternmed.2020.4130

6. Clarke KEN, Jones JM, Deng Y, et al. Seroprevalence of infection-induced SARS-CoV-2 antibodies - United States, September 2021-February 2022. *MMWR Morb Mortal Wkly Rep*. 2022 Apr 29;71(17):606–608. doi:10.15585/mmwr.mm7117e3

7. Worldometer. Coronavirus cases. Available at: https://www.worldometers.info/coronavirus/country/us. Accessed April 11, 2023.

8. DeMartino JK, Swallow E, Goldschmidt D, et al. Direct health care costs associated with COVID-19 in the United States. *J Manag Care Spec Pharm*. 2022 Sep;28(9):936–947. doi:10.18553/jmcp.2022.22050

9. Kaiser Family Foundation. Cost of COVID-19 hospital admissions among people with private health coverage. Available at: https://www.kff.org/coronavirus-covid-19/issue-brief/cost-of-covid-19-hospital-admissions-among-people-with-private-health-coverage/. Accessed February 16, 2023.

10. Institute for Progress. Weighing the cost of the pandemic. Available at: https://progress.institute/weighing-the-cost-of-the-pandemic/. Accessed February 16, 2023.

11. Zhai P, Ding Y, Wu X, Long J, Zhong Y, Li Y. The epidemiology, diagnosis and treatment of COVID-19. *Int J Antimicrob Agents*. 2020 May;55(5):105955. doi:10.1016/j.ijantimicag.2020.105955

12. Hu B, Guo H, Zhou P, Shi ZL. Characteristics of SARS-CoV-2 and COVID-19. Nat Rev Microbiol. 2021 Mar;19(3):141–154. doi:10.1038/s41579-020-00459-7. Epub 2020 Oct 6. Erratum in: *Nat Rev Microbiol*. 2022 May;20(5):315.

13. Infectious Disease Society of America. Understanding risk for severe COVID-19. Available at: https://www.idsociety.org/covid-19-real-time-learning-network/disease-manifestations--complications/understanding-risk-for-severe-covid-19/. Accessed February 16, 2023.

14. Kaiser Family Foundation. COVID-19 cases and deaths by race/ethnicity: Current data and changes over time. San Francisco, CA: KFF. Available at: https://www.kff.org/coronavirus-covid-19/issue-brief/covid-19-cases-and-deaths-by-race-ethnicity-current-data-and-changes-over-time/. Accessed February 16, 2023.

15. Kaiser Family Foundation. Latest data on covid-19 vaccinations by race/ethnicity. San Francisco, CA: KFF. Available at: https://www.kff.org/coronavirus-covid-19/issue-brief/latest-data-on-covid-19-vaccinations-by-race-ethnicity/. Accessed February 16, 2023.

16. U.S. Department of Health and Human Services. Clinical spectrum. Washington, DC: HHS. Available at: https://www.covid19treatmentguidelines.nih.gov/overview/clinical-spectrum/. Accessed February 16, 2023.

17. Struyf T, Deeks JJ, Dinnes J, Takwoingi Y, Davenport C, Leeflang MM, Spijker R, Hooft L, Emperador D, Domen J, Tans A, Janssens S, Wickramasinghe D, Lannoy V, Horn SRA, Van den Bruel A; Cochrane COVID-19 Diagnostic Test Accuracy Group. Signs and symptoms to determine if a patient presenting in primary care or hospital outpatient settings has COVID-19. *Cochrane Database Syst Rev*. 2022 May 20;5(5):CD013665. doi:10.1002/14651858.CD013665.pub3

18. Centers for Disease Control and Prevention. Overview of testing for SARS-COV-2, the virus that causes COVID-19. Atlanta, GA: CDC. Available at: https://www.cdc.gov/coronavirus/2019-ncov/hcp/testing-overview.html. Accessed February 16, 2023.

19. U.S. Department of Health and Human Services. Clinical management of adults summary. Washington, DC: HHS. Available at: https://www.covid19treatmentguidelines.nih.gov/management/clinical-management-of-adults/clinical-management-of-adults-summary/?utm_source=site&utm_medium=home&utm_campaign=highlights. Accessed February 16, 2023.

20. Infectious Disease Society of America. Rapid testing. Arlington, VA: IDSA. Available at: https://www.idsociety.org/covid-19-real-time-learning-network/diagnostics/rapid-testing/. Accessed February 16, 2023.

21. Cascella M, Rajnik M, Aleem A, et al. Features, Evaluation, and Treatment of Coronavirus (COVID-19) [Updated 2023 Jan 9]. In: StatPearls [Internet]. Treasure Island (FL): StatPearls Publishing; 2023 Jan.

22. Centers for Disease Control and Prevention. Guidance for antigen testing for SARS-COV-2 for healthcare providers testing individuals in the community. Atlanta, GA: CDC. Available at: https://stacks.cdc.gov/view/cdc/115045. Accessed February 16, 2023.

23. Infectious Disease Society of America. Covid-19 Guideline, part 1: Treatment and management. Arlington, VA: IDSA. Available at: https://www.idsociety.org/practice-guideline/covid-19-guideline-treatment-and-management/. Accessed February 16, 2023.

24. Administration for Strategic Preparedness and Response. Expanding access to covid 19 therapeutics. Available at: https://aspr.hhs.gov/COVID-19/Therapeutics/updates/Pages/default.aspx. Accessed August 9, 2024.
25. LumiraDx. LumiraDx COVID-19 antigen test. COVID-19 SARS-CoV-2 Antigen Test | (US). Available at: https://www.lumiradx.com/us-en/test-menu/antigen-test. Accessed February 16, 2023.
26. BD Veritor. Fact sheet for healthcare providers coronavirus TM system. Available at: https://bdveritor.bd.com/content/dam/bdveritor/pdfs/BDVeritor_COVID-19_HCP-FactSheet31Mar21.pdf. Accessed February 16, 2023.
27. Quidel. HCP fact sheet–Quidel. Available at: https://www.quidel.com/sites/default/files/product/documents/FS2037404EN00.pdf. Accessed February 16, 2023.
28. Cepheid. Xpert® Xpress SARS-COV-2 has received FDA Emergency Use Authorization. Available at: https://www.cepheid.com/coronavirus. Accessed February 16, 2023.

CHAPTER 9

Human Immunodeficiency Virus

Alexis Page, PharmD, BCACP

Key Points

- Human immunodeficiency virus (HIV) is the virus that causes Acquired Immunodeficiency Syndrome (AIDS) a manageable, chronic disease that can be prevented with pre-exposure prophylaxis (PrEP).
- All adolescents and adults should be screened for HIV at least once in their lifetime and more often if risk factors are present.
- There are several CLIA-waived rapid HIV POCTs available to screen for HIV in community and ambulatory care settings.
- PrEP should be offered to individuals at high risk of HIV acquisition and to those who request PrEP regardless of indication.
- PrEP is available in both oral and injectable formulations.
- Follow-up is critical for successful reduction of HIV transmission risk and should occur every 3 months.

The human immunodeficiency virus (HIV) was identified in the 1980s as the virus responsible for causing acquired immunodeficiency syndrome (AIDS). This new virus spurred a global epidemic, with 337 AIDS cases reported in the United States by the end of 1981 alone.[1] Over 40 years later, this once terminal diagnosis has become a chronic, manageable, disorder with considerably greater life expectancy.

There are three types of HIV infections, HIV-1, HIV-2, and HIV-1/HIV-2 dual infection. HIV-1 is the most common type of HIV infection worldwide, with HIV-2 infection occurring predominantly in West African areas.[2] The most common methods of HIV transmission include anal or vaginal sex; sharing needles, syringes or other devices used to inject drugs; and perinatal transmission, where a mother transmits HIV to her child during pregnancy, birth or breastfeeding.[3] Risk factors for HIV exposure include having condomless anal or vaginal sex, concomitant sexually transmitted infection (STI), harmful use of alcohol and drugs while engaging in sexual behavior, sharing needles or other devices to inject drugs, and accidental needlesticks, particularly in health care.[4]

As of 2021, there are roughly 38.4 million individuals globally living with HIV, with the highest prevalence (95%) in individuals ages 15 years and older. Of these 38.4 million people, 25.6 million reside in African Regions.[5] That same year, it was estimated that 1.5 million people were newly diagnosed with HIV, a 32% decline in new HIV infections since 2010.[6] In the United States, approximately 1.2 million people are HIV positive, with 34,800 new diagnoses in 2019, an 8% decline from 2015. In 2020, 71% of new cases were diagnosed in gay and bisexual men and men who have sex with men (MSM), and 26% and 21% of new cases were diagnosed in Black/African American and Hispanic/Latino populations, respectively.[7]

Pharmacists have a role in the prevention, diagnosis, and treatment of HIV.[8] This chapter will focus on POCT with regards to the prevention and diagnosis of HIV in community and ambulatory pharmacy settings.

Clinical Presentation

The clinical presentation of HIV infection varies based on the progression of the illness, which is divided into 3 stages. The first stage, also known as acute HIV infection, presents 2 to 4 weeks after initial infection as flu-like symptoms, including fever, rash, chills, night sweats, muscle aches, sore throat, and fatigue.[9,10] Two-thirds of individuals typically present symptoms of acute infection; however, one-third of people are asymptomatic in the first stage and may be unaware they are infected.[9] If symptoms do present, they may last between days and weeks before eventually subsiding. HIV is most contagious during the first stage of HIV, when there is a large amount of HIV in the blood within the first few months of being infected. However, many are unaware of their status during this time, highlighting the importance of routine testing.[9]

The second stage, also known as chronic HIV infection or clinical latency, occurs when HIV is still actively replicating but at much lower levels. People are typically asymptomatic, and the infection may remain latent for 5 to 10 years, or longer, without treatment.[9,10] If left untreated, the infection will eventually cause the individual's immune system to weaken, transitioning the individual into stage 3, also known as AIDS. Those who receive treatment for HIV may never progress to stage 3 and can suppress viral loads sufficiently to prevent the spread of HIV to sexual partners.[9,10]

As the HIV-infected person moves from stage 2 into stage 3, their CD4 cell counts will decrease, allowing HIV viral loads to increase. AIDS is typically diagnosed when CD4 counts drop below 200 cells/mm, or when the individual contracts opportunistic infections to which only severely immunocompromised people would be susceptible.[11] Symptoms of AIDS include rapid weight loss, recurring fever or profuse night sweats, extreme fatigue, swollen lymph nodes, skin rashes, diarrhea, and sores in or near the mouth, anus or genitals.[9,10]

The role of the community and ambulatory care pharmacist performing HIV POCT focuses on prevention and referral for further evaluation. When performing POCT for HIV detection, the pharmacist should monitor for any signs or symptoms of any of the 3 stages of HIV. Flu-like symptoms are not a contraindication to conducting HIV POCT, although the patient should be counseled on the window period for HIV POCT if the patient is symptomatic and receives a negative test result.[12] The window period is the time between HIV exposure and the time that HIV may first be detected in the body and is dependent on which POCT is used.[12] Signs and symptoms of AIDS are not a contraindication of HIV POCT, although the patient should be referred for further evaluation regardless of test result.

Point-of-Care Testing

Due to the ability for the virus to lay dormant for years after initial infection, it is estimated that 1 in 8 people with HIV are unaware that they are infected.[13] CDC recommends HIV screening for all people ages 13 to 64 years old at least once as part of their routine care, and those at higher risk should be tested more frequently.[13] The U.S. Preventive Services Task Force (USPSTF) recommends screening for HIV in people ages 15 to 65 years old and pregnant persons, although no optimal interval has been defined.[14] Repeat screening is appropriate for those with additional risk factors.[14,28]

Three different types of HIV tests are available, with antibody (Ab) and antibody/antigen (Ab/Ag) tests being most common in outpatient settings (Table 9–1).

Table 9–1. Types of HIV tests available[12,15–17]

Type of test	Mechanism of action	Window period	Clinical pearls
Nucleic acid test (NAT)	Detect presence of virus in the blood	10 to 33 days	• Consider for those who have had recent exposure • Requires venipuncture, no POCT available
Antibody (Ab) test	Detect IgM and/or IgG antibodies	23 to 90 days	• May be conducted with blood or saliva • Often are rapid tests, some tests yield results in minutes • Timing of the test after exposure is crucial
Antibody and antigen (Ab/Ag) test	Detect IgM and IgG antibodies and antigen p24	Lab Test: 18 to 45 days Rapid Test: 18 to 90 days	• Rapid tests may not be as sensitive as lab test

Key: POCT, point-of-care test.

Sites performing rapid HIV testing must obtain a certificate of waiver under the Clinical Laboratory Improvement Amendment (CLIA) to use CLIA-waived POCTs.[18] No CLIA-waived NATs are available, so rapid HIV testing is typically performed with Ab or Ab/Ag tests. Facilities using rapid Ab HIV tests are also required to have a quality assurance plan to ensure that testing is performed correctly and results are accurate, with the goal of ensuring the safety of the individual and others.[18] Blood is the preferred sample source for early HIV detection, because tests using blood are more sensitive than those using oral fluid; however, oral fluid can be used for certain tests, including self-tests.[15] See Table 9–2 below.

Table 9–2. CLIA-waived rapid HIV POCTs[17,19-25]

Type of test	Test name	Manufacturer	Sample source	Result time	Cost
Ab/Ag	Alere Determine HIV-1/2 Ag/Ab Combo[24]	Abbott	Whole blood	20 minutes	$$
Ab	HIV-1/2 STAT-PAK[19]	Chembio Diagnostic	Whole blood	15 minutes	$
Ab	OraQuick Advance Rapid[23] HIV-1/2	OraSure Technologies	Oral fluid, whole blood	20 minutes	$$
Ab	Sure Check HIV-1/2[20]	Chembio Diagnostic	Whole blood	15 minutes	$
Ab	DPP HIV-1/2 Assay[21]	Chembio Diagnostic	Oral fluid, whole blood	10–40 minutes	$
Ab	bioLytical INSTI HIV-1/HIV-2 Antibody Test[22]	bioLytical	Whole blood	<2 minutes	$$$
Ab	Uni-Gold Recombigen HIV-1/2[25]	Trinity Biotech	Whole blood	10 minutes	$$

The preferred method of testing for HIV in the context of preexposure prophylaxis (PrEP) treatment is either laboratory diagnostic testing of a whole-blood sample or a rapid, FDA-approved, POC fingerstick Ab/Ag blood test. Tests that use oral fluid should not be used to screen for HIV infection because they are less sensitive for detection of recent infection.[27]

Pharmacists in community and ambulatory care settings are well positioned to screen individuals for HIV and assist them in obtaining further care if appropriate.[8] A positive POCT in a community or ambulatory pharmacy setting does not confirm an HIV diagnosis; a patient with a positive HIV POCT should be referred to a HCP for a follow-up test.[8,26] Prior to starting HIV POCT in a community or ambulatory care setting, HCPs should ensure that policies and procedures are established for training staff members to assist those who test positive with obtaining care and preventive services.[8] Those who test negative for HIV should be counseled on risk factors for contracting HIV and the benefits and risks of PrEP medication.

Treatment

All patients who test positive for HIV should receive HIV treatment.[27] If a patient tests positive for HIV in a community or ambulatory care pharmacy setting, the patient should be referred to an HCP who can order confirmatory testing and prescribe treatment if appropriate.[8,15]

For those who test negative for HIV, the HCP should determine if the patient is a candidate for PrEP medication.[26] PrEP medication may be initiated with the goal of preventing HIV infection if a patient has been knowingly or unknowingly exposed, and all sexually active persons should be counseled on the role of PrEP in terms of HIV transmission.[26] PrEP should be offered to those at substantial risk of HIV exposure, including:

- Persons who have had anal or vaginal sex in the past 6 months with an HIV+ partner with an unknown or detectable viral load
- Persons who have had condomless anal or vaginal sex in the past 6 months with at least one person with unknown HIV status
- Persons who have had a bacterial STI in the past 6 months:
    - MSM: chlamydia, syphilis, or gonorrhea
    - Men who have sex with women (MSW) and women who have sex with men (WSM): syphilis or gonorrhea
- Persons who have shared drug injection equipment in the past 6 months.[26]

Some patients may not be comfortable disclosing their sexual history or drug use due to fear of being stigmatized. Therefore, PrEP should also be initiated to patients who request it, regardless of lack of indication or documented risk behaviors.[26] Other considerations for PrEP indication and eligibility include screening for alcohol use disorder or use of illicit non-injectable drugs, as these substances may impact sexual risk behavior, renal health, and medication adherence.[26]

Certain STI tests, such as those for gonorrhea, chlamydia, and syphilis, are recommended at regular intervals for specific populations. Gonorrhea tests are recommended for all sexually active adults receiving PrEP at the time of initiation, whereas they are recommended quarterly for MSM and semi-annually women. Chlamydia screenings are recommended for all women at the time of PrEP initiation and annually. Lastly, syphilis screenings are recommended at the time of PrEP initiation and semi-annually for both men and women receiving PrEP medication.[26]

In addition to HIV and STI testing, routine laboratory testing results should be evaluated prior to prescribing PrEP. Renal function should be assessed because reduced renal function can be a contraindication for PrEP therapy. Patients should be screened for hepatitis B (HBV) infection prior to receiving PrEP therapy; if the test is positive, PrEP should be initiated in consultation with an HBV treatment expert. Patients who receive tenofovir alafenamide (TAF) should have their lipid profile reviewed upon initiation and annually for rising triglyceride and cholesterol levels.[26] Table 9–3 summarizes the screening guidelines for oral PrEP candidates and recipients.

Table 9-3. Routine testing recommendations for oral[a] PrEP recipients[26]

Test	Screening intervals	CDC required or recommended	Target populations
HIV Test	Initial, then every 3 months (oral) or every 2 months (injection)	Required	All patients beginning and receiving PrEP
eCrCl	Initial, then every 6 to 12 months, depending on age and renal function	Required	All patients beginning and receiving PrEP
Hep B serology	Initial	Recommended	All patients beginning and receiving PrEP
Lipid panel	Initial, then annually	Recommended	Descovy recipients
Gonorrhea	Initial, then quarterly (MSM) or semi-annually (women)	Recommended	All patients beginning and receiving PrEP
Chlamydia	Initial, then quarterly (MSM) or semi-annually (women)	Recommended	All patients beginning and receiving PrEP
Syphilis	Initial, then semi-annually	Recommended	All patients beginning PrEP

[a]Slight deviations in screening intervals for those who receive cabotegravir injections. For more information, review www.cdc.gov/hiv/pdf/risk/prep/cdc-hiv-prep-guidelines-2021.pdf.

A documented negative HIV test result is required prior to PrEP initiation and should be repeated every 3 months for those who are receiving oral PrEP therapy or every 2 months for those receiving PrEP via injection.[26] A negative HIV test should be documented within the first week of initial PrEP prescribing. Renal function must also be assessed to safely initiate PrEP therapy. Three medications are approved by the U.S. Food and Drug Administration (FDA) for HIV PrEP: emtricitabine (F) in combination with tenofovir disoproxil fumarate (TDF), F in combination with TAF, and cabotegravir (Table 9-4).

Table 9-4. FDA-approved PrEP therapy[28-30]

Brand name	Generic	Dose	Route	Frequency	Common adverse effects
Truvada	F/TDF	200 mg/ 300 mg	Oral	CrCl >50 mL/min: Every 24 hours CrCl 30 to 49 L/min: Every 48 hours CrCl <30mL/min: Do not administer	Headache, abdominal pain, weight loss
Descovy	F/TAF	200 mg/ 25 mg	Oral	CrCl >30 mL/min: Every 24 hours CrCl <30 mL/min: Do not administer	Diarrhea, nausea, abdominal pain, fatigue, headache
Apretude	Cabotegravir	600 mg	IM	Every 2 months	Induration/nodule at injection site, injection site reaction, headache

F/TDF is the most prescribed medication for PrEP and is typically prescribed once daily, depending on renal function. Cabotegravir injections may be initiated with or without oral lead-in. If oral lead-in is preferred, the patient should take 30 mg cabotegravir once daily for at least 28 days, then receive a cabotegravir injection on the last day of lead-in therapy or within three days after.[26]

For some patients, delaying PrEP initiation may be harmful if the patient encounters barriers to returning to the clinical site or if the patient has high-risk behaviors that would increase risk of infection between the time when the HIV test was conducted and when PrEP is initiated. For this reason, PrEP may be initiated on the same day when the HIV test is conducted if the following conditions are met:

1. Conduct POCT HIV ab/ag test
2. Conduct POCT for creatinine
    a. May draw blood for laboratory creatinine if same-day creatinine test results are not available
3. Offer assistance for health insurance enrollment, medication co-payment or assistance programs for those who are eligible
4. Provide rapid follow-up for those whose laboratory test results indicate HIV infection or renal dysfunction
5. Schedule follow-up appointments
6. HCP has the ability to prescribe and dispense oral PrEP medication or administer injectable PrEP medication

PrEP should not be initiated on the same day as the HIV test if the patient is ambivalent about starting PrEP, presents with signs or symptoms and sexual history of possible acute HIV infection or has a past medical history of renal disease or associated conditions, such as diabetes or hypertension. Patients should also be able to pay for PrEP when prescribed, either through insurance or a patient assistance program. Same-day PrEP initiation is not appropriate for those who have had a very recent possible HIV exposure, those who do not have a confirmed method of contact for follow-up or those with mental health conditions that would impact their ability to be adherent to the medication regimen and follow-up appointments.[26]

At the time of PrEP initiation, the patient should be counseled on the medication dosage and schedule, common adverse effects, the relationship of adherence to the efficacy of PrEP, signs and symptoms of acute HIV infection, and action steps if those present. The patient should also be counseled on the recommended follow-up intervals. It is recommended that HCPs provide follow-up with PrEP patients every 3 months to provide repeat HIV testing, screen for signs and symptoms of acute HIV infection, assess adherence, and refill the PrEP prescription. Additional STI and renal function screenings are recommended at various intervals, which reinforce the importance of regular follow-up with PrEP patients.[26]

Patient Cases

Patient Case 9–1 SOAP Note

Collect	Chief Complaint
Subjective	A 31-year-old African American man (AC) presents to the pharmacy requesting an HIV test and PrEP consultation.
Objective	Past medical history (PMH)
	AC presents to the pharmacy requesting an HIV test and education about PrEP. He states that he is a gay man who is interested in beginning PrEP. AC had taken Truvada previously for 6 months in 2019, but he stopped when he entered into a monogamous relationship with his former partner. AC is no longer in a monogamous relationship as of January 2022 and wants to protect himself from HIV. AC has anonymous sex with multiple partners and tries to always wear a condom, but he admits that he does not wear a condom 100% of the time. AC had one occurrence of gonorrhea infection in May 2022, which was resolved with medication. At that time, AC received a negative HIV test. AC does not use illicit drugs aside from daily marijuana use. AC's last sexual encounter was 6 weeks ago with an anonymous partner who wore a condom. AC states that he is adherent to medications that are prescribed and missed on average one dose of Truvada per month when last prescribed. AC did not bring copies of his most recent lab work from his PCP but was able to log into his chart on his phone and provide the most recent lab values.
	Attention deficit/hyperactivity disorder
	Gonorrhea—2022, resolved
	Social history (SH)
	Lives alone, employed as a software developer, has local family support
	Has been sexually active previously with eight partners
	Illicit drugs: uses marijuana regularly, began at age 25, no other history of drug use
	Tobacco: never smoker
	Alcohol: only drinks socially
	Insurance: commercial insurance through employer
	Family History
	Mother—alive, age 59, HTN, GERD, hypothyroidism
	Father—alive, age 63, T2DM
	Sister—alive, 33, no chronic conditions
	Allergies: None
	Medications
	Vyvanse 50 mg once daily for ADHD
	Immunizations
	Fluarix: 10/28/2022
	Heplisav-B: 08/05/2015, 09/30/2015, 01/10/2016
	Jynneos: 9/15/2022, 10/20/2022
	Temperature: 98.5°F; pulse: 78 bpm; respiratory rate (RR): 18 breaths/minute; BP: 126/72 mm HG; O2 saturation: 99%; height: 73 in; weight: 190 lbs
	HIV rapid test: negative (-)

Patient Case 9–1 SOAP Note cont'd

	Laboratory test results from 11/16/2022 PCP visit: CrCl: >60 mL/min Syphilis: negative (-) Gonorrhea: negative (-) Chlamydia: negative (-) Total cholesterol: 194 mg/dL LDL: 92 mg/dL HDL: 40 mg/dL Triglycerides: 172 mg/dL HCV antibody: non-reactive (-)
Assess	AC is an HIV-negative African American male who would benefit from PrEP medication. His risk factors for HIV exposure include occasional condomless sex, sex with multiple partners with unknown HIV status, and recent STI infection, although the infection occurred more than 6 months ago. AC does not have any signs or symptoms of acute HIV infection, was not recently exposed to HIV, and has sufficient renal function (CrCl >60 mL/min) to begin PrEP therapy.
Plan	Initiate Truvada 200 mg/300 mg once daily for 90 days. Schedule follow-up in 3 months to monitor for signs and symptoms of acute HIV infection and adverse effects and evaluate medication adherence. Patient should be counseled on the importance of medication adherence, s/sx of acute HIV infection, time to achieve protection from daily oral PrEP and the importance of follow-up.
Implement	AC was prescribed Truvada once daily for 90 days, with no refills. AC can afford Truvada with his private insurance plan with a co-pay of zero dollars. AC was counseled on: S/sx of acute HIV infection: fever, rash, chills, night sweats, muscle aches, sore throat, and fatigue Truvada adverse effects Importance of adherence Truvada does not completely eliminate the risk of acquiring HIV and dose not reduce the risk of acquiring STIs Safe sex practices, such as condoms and avoiding using illicit drugs that could increase high-risk sexual behaviors
Monitor/ Follow-Up	Three-month follow-up scheduled: Assess HIV status Assess adverse effects and advise on how to manage Assess STI symptoms and HIV risk behavior Assess medication adherence

Patient Case 9–2 SOAP Note

Collect	Chief Complaint
Subjective	A 26-year-old pregnant Caucasian woman presents to the pharmacy requesting an HIV test.
Objective	Past Medical History (PMH)
	DL is a Caucasian woman who states that she was referred to your practice by a community health worker since she is a sex worker and wants to protect herself from HIV. She is roughly 5 months pregnant, but she has not seen an HCP since she does not have insurance. She states that she heard that PrEP was free and wants to begin treatment to reduce her chances of contracting HIV. She thinks the number of sexual partners she has had in the past month is between 15 and 20, and she states that she sometimes does not use condoms when having sex. DL states that she is just getting over COVID and has lingering fatigue, chills, muscle aches and a sore throat.
	Temperature: 97.5°F; pulse: 98 bpm; RR: 16 breaths/minute; BP: 144/90 mm HG; O_2 saturation: 97%; height: 64 in; weight: 155 lbs
	HIV rapid test: positive (+)
Assess	DL is a 26-year-old pregnant woman with possible acute HIV infection. Her rapid HIV test is positive and DL is presenting with s/sx of acute HIV infection, such as fatigue, chills, muscle aches and a sore throat, which may or may not be COVID-related. DL would benefit from confirmatory HIV testing and additional care.
Plan	Provide test result to DL and refer her to the nearest local health department (LHD) to receive confirmatory laboratory HIV testing, prenatal care, and enrollment into Medicaid.
Implement	DL was educated on her rapid HIV test result and the importance of additional care. DL was referred to the nearest LHD and was provided their address, directions, and telephone number. The local health department was notified of referral via fax.
Monitor/ Follow-Up	Telephone call scheduled in a week with patient to follow-up on LHD referral.

Conclusion

- HIV is a manageable, chronic disease that can be prevented with PrEP.
- All adolescents and adults should be screened for HIV at least once in their lifetime and more often if risk factors are present.
- There are several CLIA-waived rapid HIV POCTs available to screen for HIV in community and ambulatory care settings.
- PrEP should be offered to individuals at high risk of HIV acquisition and to those who request PrEP regardless of indication.
- PrEP is available in both oral and injectable formulations.
- Follow-up is critical for successful reduction of HIV transmission risk and should occur every 3 months.

References

1. U.S. Department of Health and Human Services. A Timeline of HIV and AIDS. Washington, DC: HHS. Available at: https://www.hiv.gov/hiv-basics/overview/history/hiv-and-aids-timeline/#year-1981. Accessed March 26, 2023.

2. U.S. Department of Health and Human Services. Guidelines for the use of antiretroviral agents in adults and adolescents with HIV. Washington, DC: HHS. Available at: https://clinicalinfo.hiv.gov/en/guidelines/hiv-clinical-guidelines-adult-and-adolescent-arv/hiv-2-infection. Accessed April 2, 2023.

3. Centers for Disease Control and Prevention. Ways HIV can be transmitted. Atlanta, GA: CDC. Available at: https://www.cdc.gov/hiv/basics/hiv-transmission/ways-people-get-hiv.html. Accessed March 12, 2023.

4. World Health Organization. HIV. Geneva, Switzerland: WHO. Available at: https://www.who.int/news-room/fact-sheets/detail/hiv-aids. Accessed March 11, 2023.

5. World Health Organization. HIV. Geneva, Switzerland: WHO. Available at: https://www.who.int/data/gho/data/themes/hiv-aids. Accessed March 26, 2023.

6. U.S. Department of Health and Human Services. The Global HIV/AIDS Epidemic. Global Statistics. Available at: https://www.hiv.gov/hiv-basics/overview/data-and-trends/global-statistics/. Accessed March 11, 2023.

7. U.S. Department of Health and Human Services. U.S. Statistics. Available at: https://www.hiv.gov/hiv-basics/overview/data-and-trends/statistics/. Accessed March 11, 2023.

8. McCree DH, Byrd KK, Johnston A, et al. Role for Pharmacists in the "Ending the HIV Epidemic: A Plan for America" Initiative. *Public Health Rep.* 2020 Sept-Oct; 135(5): 547–554. doi:10.1177/0033354920941184

9. U.S. Department of Health and Human Services. Symptoms of HIV. Available at: https://www.hiv.gov/hiv-basics/overview/about-hiv-and-aids/symptoms-of-hiv/. Accessed March 26, 2023.

10. Centers for Disease Control and Prevention. About HIV. Atlanta, GA: CDC. Available at: https://www.cdc.gov/hiv/about/. Accessed March 26, 2023.

11. Centers for Disease Control and Prevention. AIDS and Opportunistic Infections. Atlanta, GA: CDC. Available at: https://www.cdc.gov/hiv/about/index.html. Accessed March 26, 2023.

12. Centers for Disease Control and Prevention. Getting Tested for HIV. Atlanta, GA: CDC. Available at: https://www.cdc.gov/hiv/testing/. Accessed March 26, 2023.

13. Centers for Disease Control and Prevention. Screening for HIV. Atlanta, GA: CDC. Available at: https://www.cdc.gov/hiv/clinicians/screening/index.html. Accessed March 26, 2023.

14. U.S. Prevention Services Task Force Recommendation Statement. Screening for HIV Infection. *JAMA.* 2019;321(23):2326–2336. doi: 10.1001/jama.2019.6587

15. Centers for Disease Control and Prevention. Implementing HIV Testing in Nonclinical Settings. Atlanta, GA: CDC. Available at: https://www.cdc.gov/hiv/pdf/testing/CDC_HIV_Implementing_HIV_Testing_in_Nonclinical_Settings.pdf. Accessed March 26, 2023.

16. Centers for Disease Control and Prevention. HIV Testing. Atlanta, GA: CDC. Available at: https://www.cdc.gov/hiv/testing/index.html. Updated 6/9/2022. Accessed March 26, 2023.

17. Centers for Disease Control and Prevention. FDA-approved HIV tests. Atlanta, GA: CDC. Available at: https://www.cdc.gov/hiv/partners/testing/laboratory-tests.html. Accessed March 26, 2023.

18. Centers for Disease Control and Prevention. CLIA Certificate of Waiver. Atlanta, GA: CDC. Available at: https://www.cdc.gov/hiv/partners/testing/nonclinical/clia.html. Updated 12/15/2021. Accessed March 26, 2023.

19. Chembio Diagnostic Systems, Inc. HIV 1/2 STAT-PAK™ Assay [package insert]. Available at: https://www.fda.gov/media/73233/download. Accessed March 26, 2023.

20. Chembio Diagnostic Systems, Inc. Sure Check HIV 1/2 Assay [package insert]. Available at: https://www.fda.gov/media/73217/download. Accessed March 26, 2023.

21. Chembio Diagnostic Systems, Inc. DPP HIV 1/2 Assay [package insert]. Available at: https://www.fda.gov/media/84916/download. Accessed March 26, 2023.

22. bioLytical Laboratories, Inc. INSTI HIV-1/HIV-2 Antibody Test Kit [package insert]. Available at: https://www.fda.gov/media/79719/download. Accessed March 26, 2023.

23. OraSure Technologies, Inc. OraQuick Advance Rapid HIV-1/2 Antibody Test [package insert]. Available at: https://www.fda.gov/media/73607/download. Accessed March 26, 2023.

24. Abbott Diagnostics Scarborough, Inc. HIV-1/2 Ag/Ab COMBO [package insert]. Available at: https://www.fda.gov/media/86959/download. Accessed March 26, 2023.

25. Trinity Biotech. Uni-Gold™ Recombigen HI-1/2 [package insert]. Available at: https://www.fda.gov/media/114893/download. Accessed March 26, 2023.

26. Centers for Disease Control and Prevention, U.S. Public Health Service. Preexposure prophylaxis for the prevention of HIV infection in the United States—2021 Update: a clinical practice guideline. Atlanta, GA: CDC. Available at: https://www.cdc.gov/hiv/pdf/risk/prep/cdc-hiv-prep-guidelines-2021.pdf. Accessed March 26, 2023.

27. National Institutes of Health. HIV Treatment. Bethesda, MD: NIH. Available at: https://hivinfo.nih.gov/understanding-hiv/fact-sheets/when-start-hiv-medicines. Accessed April 1, 2023.

28. UpToDate Inc. Emtricitabine and tenofovir disoproxil fumarate oral. Facts and Comparisons online, Facts and Comparisons eAnswers online. Waltham, MA: UpToDate. Available at: https://fco.factsandcomparisons.com. Accessed April 1, 2023.

29. UpToDate Inc. Emtricitabine and tenofovir alafenamide oral. Facts and Comparisons online, Facts and Comparisons eAnswers online. Waltham, MA: UpToDate. Available at: https://fco.factsandcomparisons.com. Accessed April 1, 2023.

30. UpToDate Inc. Cabotegravir Injection. Facts and Comparisons online, Facts and Comparisons eAnswers online. Waltham, MA: UpToDate. Available at: https://fco.factsandcomparisons.com. Accessed April 1, 2023.

CHAPTER 10

Other Disorders Related to Infectious Diseases

Barbara A. Santevecchi, PharmD, BCIDP and
Lindsey M. Childs-Kean, PharmD, MPH, BCPS

Key Points

- Implementation of POCT for *H. pylori* may contribute to increased access to treatment for eradication, thereby decreasing complications associated with this infection (e.g., peptic ulcer disease, gastric cancer).
- The presence of urinary symptoms is required to differentiate urinary tract infection (UTI) from asymptomatic bacteriuria (ASB), the latter of which does not require antibiotic treatment in most patients.
- Patients presenting with complicated cystitis, pyelonephritis, or UTI with systemic signs of infection should be referred to a PCP for management.
- Most RSV infections are mild and managed with supportive care, but patients presenting with severe illness and/or those who test positive and are at risk for severe disease should be referred to a PCP for management.
- All adults should be tested for HCV at least once, and this testing can be done by POCT.
- Individuals with signs or symptoms of decompensated cirrhosis should receive a medical referral.

This chapter will review several infectious diseases that may be applicable to point-of-care (POCT) test-and-treat programs. These include Helicobacter pylori (H. pylori) infection, urinary tract infection (UTI), RSV, and HCV. A wide variety of patients may be affected by these disease states, and use of POCT and test-and-treat programs in the pharmacy setting may serve to increase access to care and support more rapid treatment initiation, when applicable.

Helicobacter pylori Infection

Helicobacter pylori (H. pylori) infection is a common, chronic bacterial infection that affects many millions of people worldwide.[1] The estimated global prevalence of H. pylori infection is approximately 50%, and wide variability is observed based on geographic location.[2] The highest frequencies of infection are seen in Asia and Central and South America, whereas the frequency in the United States is relatively lower.[1] In addition, the prevalence of infection may vary based on race or ethnicity, with the highest rates reported among Hispanic and African American populations.[1,2] Most people acquire H. pylori during childhood. Some of the risk factors associated with infection include low socioeconomic status, crowded living conditions, contamination of food or water supplies, poor sanitation, a high number of siblings, and having an infected parent.[1,2] Transmission occurs most commonly via the fecal-oral or oral-oral routes through consumption of contaminated food or water.[2] H. pylori infection may contribute to the development of gastritis, dyspepsia, peptic ulcer disease, or other gastrointestinal diseases, including gastric cancer.[2]

Clinical Presentation

The majority of people infected with H. pylori are asymptomatic and will remain without symptoms during their lifetime.[3] Patients with peptic ulcer disease resulting from H. pylori infection may present with epigastric pain, which is often described as a burning or gnawing sensation.[3] Less common symptoms of H. pylori infection include nausea, vomiting, and loss of appetite.[3] Alarm symptoms that require evaluation by a PCP include unexplained weight loss, severe abdominal pain or presence of an abdominal mass, dysphagia, odynophagia, vomiting, jaundice or gastrointestinal bleeding.[4] POCT may be considered in patients younger than 60 years old with uninvestigated dyspepsia who do not have alarm symptoms.[1]

Diagnosis

Indications for testing to identify H. pylori infection are provided in the American College of Gastroenterology guidelines and included in Table 10-1. Testing is not recommended for patients with symptoms typical of gastroesophageal reflux disease (GERD) who do not have a history of peptic ulcer disease. Histologic diagnosis through endoscopic sampling of gastric tissue has high sensitivity and specificity reported above 95%.[5] In patients with indications for testing and without an indication for endoscopy (including no alarm symptoms as listed above), noninvasive testing may be considered.[5]

Table 10-1. Indications for *H. pylori* testing[1,5]

Active or history of peptic ulcer disease (PUD), unless *H. pylori* has been eradicated
Low-grade gastric mucosa-associated lymphoid tissue (MALT) lymphoma
History of endoscopic resection of early gastric cancer
Uninvestigated dyspepsia
Long-term aspirin or NSAID use
Unexplained iron deficiency anemia
Immune thrombocytopenia in adults
To document eradication following completion of treatment for *H. pylori* infection

Physical Assessment

Most patients with *H. pylori* infection are asymptomatic, and therefore may not seek testing. Patients who request testing for *H. pylori* may present with dyspepsia and/or epigastric pain.[4] POCT for *H. pylori* requires collection of a blood sample to perform serologic testing.[4]

Point-of-Care Testing

Serological tests are POCTs available for *H. pylori* detection that may be implemented in the pharmacy setting. These tests detect the presence of *H. pylori* immunoglobulin G (IgG) in the serum, but they cannot be used to distinguish between active infection and past infection.[4] In addition, serological testing does not require discontinuation of proton pump inhibitor (PPI) therapy, unlike some other noninvasive testing methods (e.g., urea breath test or stool antigen test).[4] Example brands of serological tests include the Polymedco Poly stat® *H. pylori* test (result available within 10 minutes) and Accutest® *H. pylori* test (result available within 3 to 7 minutes).[6,7]

Treatment

All patients with a positive test indicating active infection with *H. pylori* should be offered treatment.[1] The goals of treatment include resolution of symptoms, eradication of the pathogen and prevention of complications of infection such as gastric cancer.[1] A guideline-recommended first-line treatment regimen for *H. pylori* infection in areas where macrolide resistance is below 15% includes a combination of twice-daily clarithromycin, amoxicillin and a PPI for 14 days.[1] For patients with prior exposure to macrolides, those who reside in areas where macrolide resistance exceeds 15%, or those with a true penicillin allergy, a four-drug regimen consisting of bismuth subsalicylate, tetracycline, metronidazole and a PPI for 10 to 14 days is recommended.[1] Factors to be considered in the selection of a treatment regimen include prior exposure to antibiotics, allergies, potential adverse effects, drug interactions, costs, insurance coverage and availability.[5] Patients must be evaluated for clearance of infection 1 month after completion of antibiotic treatment, and serologic testing should not be used for this indication as antibodies may persist for several years following infection.[5]

Indications for Referral

Figure 10–1. Algorithm for *H. pylori* POCT[1,4]

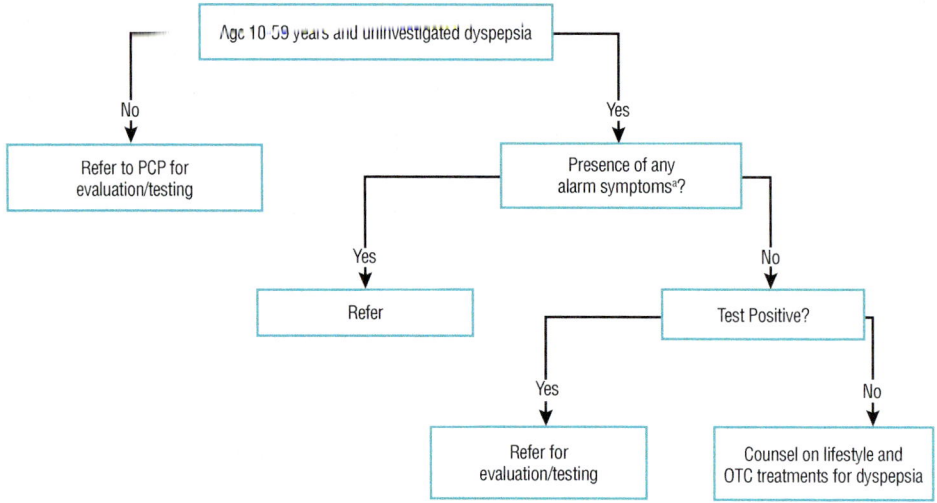

[a]Alarm symptoms: unexplained weight loss, severe abdominal pain or presence of an abdominal mass, dysphagia, odynophagia, vomiting, jaundice, or gastrointestinal bleeding.

Key: PCP, primary care physician.

An algorithm for the evaluation of patients for *H. pylori* POCTs is provided in Figure 10–1. The American College of Gastroenterology *H. pylori* guidelines state that non-endoscopic testing (such as POCT) may be considered in all patients under the age of 60 years with uninvestigated dyspepsia and without alarm symptoms (listed in Figure 10–1).[1] Patients who do not meet these criteria should be referred to a PCP to be evaluated for testing and further management. In addition, patients with a history of *H. pylori* infection should not undergo POCT using serological testing because this type of test cannot differentiate active infection from prior infection.[5] Patients who are appropriate for POCT and subsequently test positive should be referred to a PCP to receive treatment. Those who test negative should be counseled on lifestyle modifications for management of dyspepsia, such as avoidance of trigger foods, minimizing alcohol consumption, smoking cessation, and increasing exercise, as well as availability of over-the-counter medications for alleviation of symptoms, such as antacids or histamine-2 receptor antagonists.[8] Patients who experience dyspepsia that fails to respond to lifestyle modifications and over-the-counter medications should be referred to a PCP for further evaluation and management.[8]

Urinary Tract Infection

Urinary tract infections (UTIs) are the most common bacterial infections and represent one of the most frequent indications for antibiotic prescriptions, especially among women in the community setting.[9,10] There are approximately 250 million UTI cases reported each year worldwide.[11] It has been reported that about 60% of women will develop at least one UTI during their lifetime, and approximately 25% of these will experience a recurrent infection within one year.[9] UTI can be classified into two syndromes: cystitis and pyelonephritis. Cystitis refers to a lower UTI that primarily affects the bladder, whereas pyelonephritis corresponds to an upper tract infection that involves the kidneys.[9] Asymptomatic bacteriuria (ASB) is defined as the presence of bacteria in the urine, with or without pyuria, without signs or symptoms attributable to UTI.[12] It is important to distinguish UTI from ASB for proper diagnosis and management of these distinct conditions, as antibiotic treatment is not recommended for the majority of patients with ASB.[12]

UTI can be further defined as uncomplicated or complicated infection. Uncomplicated UTI refers to infection in patients who do not have structural or functional abnormalities of the urinary tract, and primarily encompasses UTI in premenopausal adult females who are otherwise healthy.[9] Complicated UTI generally refers to UTI in all other scenarios; Table 10–2 lists common factors that are associated with complicated infections. Complicated UTIs are associated with a higher risk of infection recurrence, progression, and severe outcomes.[13] While uncomplicated UTIs are mainly restricted to female patients, complicated UTIs may occur in male or female patients.[9] It is vital to classify UTI appropriately as cystitis or pyelonephritis and uncomplicated or complicated, because these designations will influence appropriate management.

Table 10–2. Common factors associated with complicated UTI[9,13]

Male sex	Ureteral stent(s)
Structural or functional abnormality of urinary tract	Nephrostomy tube(s)
Urinary stones or strictures	Pregnancy
Indwelling urinary catheter	Diabetes mellitus (especially uncontrolled)
Prostatic hypertrophy	Chronic kidney disease
Urinary tract obstruction	Immunosuppression
Neurological dysfunction (such as neurogenic bladder)	Renal transplant

Clinical presentation

It is of utmost importance to determine whether urinary symptoms are present to differentiate UTI from ASB. Symptoms consistent with cystitis include dysuria, urgency, increased urination frequency, nocturia and suprapubic pain.[9] Symptoms associated with upper urinary tract involvement consistent with pyelonephritis include flank pain, fever, nausea, vomiting, and malaise.[9] Notably, changes in urine color or odor are not specific for UTI and instead may be reflective of hydration status, consumption of certain foods, or medications.[14] Older adults may not present with typical urinary symptoms and instead may experience nonspecific symptoms, such as altered mental status.[9] It is recommended to evaluate for other etiologies besides UTI in older adult patients who present with acute mental status changes without local genitourinary symptoms or other signs of infection.[12] This strategy is suggested to avoid unnecessary exposure to antibiotics, as well as prompt clinicians to identify other potential causes of altered mental status.[12] Complications of untreated UTI may include progression of infection (such as from cystitis to pyelonephritis), urosepsis and death.[9,13]

Diagnosis

As symptoms alone are not reliable for diagnosis, the presence of UTI is confirmed by laboratory testing or POCT.[9] The procedures for such testing include collection of a urine sample to be sent for urinalysis and/or urine culture. In addition, urine dipstick testing is utilized in some practice settings to detect the presence or absence of leukocyte esterase and nitrite.[9] Leukocyte esterase indicates the presence of white blood cells in the urine, and a positive result may indicate infection or inflammation.[9] Nitrite is formed by bacteria that reduce nitrate in the urine (such as *Escherichia coli*, *Proteus* spp., and *Klebsiella* spp.).[9,15] Tests that utilize both leukocyte esterase and nitrite have a reported specificity of 82% and positive predictive value of 79% for detection of bacteria in urine.[9] It is important to correlate the presence of bacteriuria with urinary symptoms to definitively diagnose UTI.[9] The most common causative pathogen associated with UTI is *E. coli*, which is responsible for 75% to 90% of uncomplicated UTIs.[9,13] UTI may also be caused by other Enterobacterales species, such as *Klebsiella* spp., *Enterobacter* spp., *Citrobacter* spp. and *Proteus* spp., *Pseudomonas aeruginosa* (more common in complicated UTI), and gram-positive organisms such as *Enterococcus* spp. and *Staphylococcus saprophyticus* (this pathogen is especially common in young, previously healthy adult females).[9,13]

Physical Assessment

Urinary symptoms, including dysuria, urgency, increased frequency, and/or suprapubic pain, should be present in patients with UTI.[9] Some patients may experience systemic symptoms, including flank pain, fever, nausea, and vomiting, and these symptoms occur most commonly in patients with pyelonephritis.[9] Female patients who present with dysuria along with vaginal discharge or odor, pruritus, or painful intercourse and no urinary urgency or frequency should be referred for evaluation of possible vaginitis, as this constellation of symptoms is not typical for UTI.[16] POCT for diagnosis of UTI require collection of a urine sample for testing.[11]

Point-of-Care Testing

The primary POCT devices available for detection of UTI are urine dipstick tests, which utilize indicators such as a color change to report detection of leukocyte esterase and nitrites in the urine.[9] A dipstick test that is positive for nitrites is specific for UTI, but it does not have high sensitivity; therefore, a negative result does not preclude the presence of UTI.[17] False negative nitrite results may be caused by organisms that do not reduce nitrate, low nitrate diets, low urinary pH, and ingestion of vitamin C, whereas false positive results may occur due to contamination or exposure of the test to air and use of phenazopyridine.[17] Detection of leukocyte esterase by dipstick testing indicates the presence of white blood cells in the urine, or pyuria.[17] The etiologies of false negative leukocyte esterase results include glycosuria (the presence of glucose and/or other sugars in the urine), elevated specific gravity, certain medications such as nitrofurantoin or cephalexin, and use of vitamin C.[17] False positive leukocyte esterase tests may result from contamination of the test.[17] Urine dipstick tests provide rapid results and are generally inexpensive, and many are available for at-home testing to be performed by the patient.[18] A comparison of some available urine dipstick tests is provided in Table 10–3 (this table does not include all brands of urine dipstick tests available for this indication). All tests listed in Table 3 provide results within 2 minutes.[18–20] Patients or HCPs should be referred to the manufacturer instructions for each test to ensure appropriate interpretation.

Table 10-3. Examples of urine dipstick tests available for UTI detection[18-20]

Test name/brand	Price[a]	Comments
my LABBOX	$$	Virtual physician consultation included at no additional charge; insurance accepted
Uqora UTI Emergency Kit	$	Test kit includes phenazopyridine tablets and methenamine and sodium salicylate tablets; insurance not accepted
stix UTI Test	$	Subscription service available; insurance not accepted
AZO Test Strips	$	Insurance not accepted
Uristat Relief PAK	$	Phenazopyridine included; insurance not accepted

[a]Price legend: $ (1–30 dollars); $$ (30–60 dollars).

Treatment

Goals of treatment include eradication of the infecting pathogen, prevention or treatment of systemic infection, avoidance of infection recurrence, and prevention of antimicrobial resistance.[9] Table 10-4 lists treatment options for uncomplicated cystitis as recommended by the IDSA guidelines. Proper classification of infection as cystitis versus pyelonephritis and uncomplicated versus complicated UTI is important for appropriate treatment decisions. For example, patients with pyelonephritis should receive an antibiotic that reaches adequate concentrations at the site of infection in renal tissue and avoid agents that only reach therapeutic concentrations in the bladder, such as nitrofurantoin.[10] Most patients with uncomplicated cystitis will experience resolution of symptoms within several days, and one study performed in nonpregnant, adult women with uncomplicated cystitis reported a mean duration of symptoms of 3.8 days.[21]

Table 10-4. Treatment options for uncomplicated cystitis[10]

Agent and dose	Duration	Considerations
Nitrofurantoin monohydrate/macrocrystals 100 mg orally twice daily	5 days	Avoid in patients with severe renal dysfunction (creatinine clearance <30 mL/minute)
Trimethoprim/sulfamethoxazole 1 DS tablet (160/800 mg) orally twice daily	3 days	Avoid in patients with true sulfa allergy
Fosfomycin 3-gram sachet orally	1 dose	May be expensive

Uncomplicated cystitis is included in POCT test-and-treat protocols in several states. At this time, states that allow both testing and treatment for uncomplicated cystitis through pharmacist-initiated processes include Kentucky (must use state-approved protocol), Kansas (must use state-approved protocol), Idaho, and Washington State.[22,23] In addition, other states, including Florida, Arkansas, and Colorado, allow development of test-and-treat programs for minor, non-chronic conditions, which may encompass uncomplicated cystitis.[23] The scope of practice and criteria for test-and-treat programs vary by state. It is recommended that pharmacists contact their state board of pharmacy for current state-specific information.

Indications for Referral

Figure 10–2. Algorithm for UTI testing and treatment in adult patients[24]

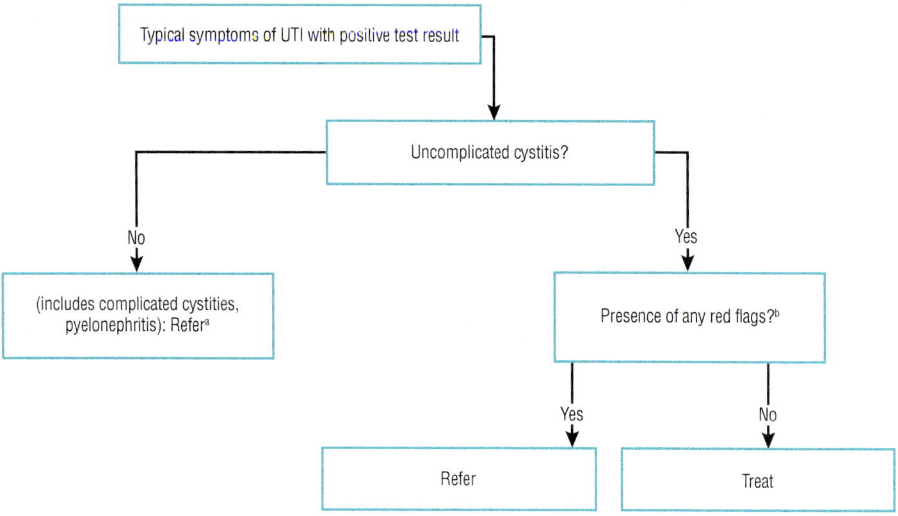

```
                    Typical symptoms of UTI with positive test result
                                         │
                                         ▼
                              Uncomplicated cystitis?
                           ┌─────────┴─────────┐
                          No                   Yes
                           │                    │
                           ▼                    ▼
              (includes complicated     Presence of any red flags?[b]
              cystities, pyelonephritis):
                      Refer[a]            ┌────┴────┐
                                         Yes        No
                                          │          │
                                          ▼          ▼
                                        Refer      Treat
```

[a]Factors associated with complicated UTI are provided in Table 10–2. Signs and symptoms that may be consistent with pyelonephritis include fever, flank pain, nausea or vomiting.
[b]Red flags include systemic signs of infection (e.g., hypotension, tachycardia, altered mental status, fever, rigors) and hematuria.

Figure 10–2 provides an algorithm to guide the appropriate testing and treatment of patients with suspected UTI. Patients who present with typical UTI symptoms (such as dysuria, urgency, increased frequency and/or suprapubic pain) and test positive for UTI should be evaluated for the presence of uncomplicated cystitis vs. complicated cystitis (criteria provided in Table 10–2) or pyelonephritis (symptoms may include fever, flank pain, nausea, or vomiting). Female patients who present with symptoms that are more consistent with vaginitis (including dysuria with vaginal discharge, odor, pruritus or painful intercourse with no urinary urgency or increased frequency) should be referred to a PCP.[16] In addition, patients who do not meet the criteria for uncomplicated cystitis should be referred to a PCP. The presence of red flags, which include systemic signs of infection (e.g., hypotension, tachycardia, altered mental status, fever, rigors) and hematuria, should prompt referral to a PCP or urgent or emergency medical services as appropriate.[24] Additional indications for PCP referral may include suspicion of the presence of a urinary tract obstruction that requires intervention by a urologist, recent urologic surgery, history of UTI caused by multidrug-resistant organism(s), worsening symptoms despite recent antibiotic therapy for the same UTI episode, and contraindications to guideline-recommended antibiotic therapy (such as allergies or severe renal dysfunction).[16] Patients should be instructed to monitor for resolution of urinary symptoms and to seek additional medical care, such as through PCP evaluation, if symptoms do not resolve or worsen with treatment.

Respiratory Syncytial Virus

RSV is a widespread viral pathogen responsible for respiratory illness in people of all ages.[25] Manifestations of infection with RSV range from asymptomatic disease to severe illness and death, especially in vulnerable populations such as infants and children who are immunosuppressed.[25,26] RSV is transmitted through inhalation or direct inoculation with viral droplets, which are produced when an infected person sneezes or coughs.[25,27] In addition, the virus can be acquired through direct contact with contaminated surfaces.[25,27] It is possible for people infected with RSV to begin spreading the virus one to two days prior to development of symptoms, and most typically remain contagious for three to eight days following infection (some infants and immunocompromised individuals may be capable of spreading the virus for up to 4 weeks post-infection).[25,27] Transmission of the virus may be prevented by frequent hand washing, avoiding close contact with those who are infected, and cleaning frequently touched surfaces.[25] The seasonality of RSV cases may vary depending on location and climate.[27] In the United States, RSV transmission typically begins in the fall and reaches a peak in winter months, with timing and severity of cases fluctuating on an annual basis.[25] Since the start of the COVID-19 pandemic in early 2020, a disruption in the seasonal patterns of RSV circulation has been seen in the United States.[25]

Most children will be infected with RSV before the age of 2 years.[25] Initial infection does not prevent subsequent infections, and reinfection with RSV is possible throughout life.[25,27] In the United States, RSV contributes to 2.1 million outpatient medical visits and up to 80,000 hospitalizations each year in children under 5 years old.[25] In addition, RSV is associated with up to 160,000 hospital admissions and up to 10,000 deaths annually in adults ≥65 years old.[25] Mortality is lower in children under 5 years old, with 100 to 300 deaths attributed to RSV each year in this age group in the United States.[25]

Clinical Presentation

A wide spectrum exists in the clinical presentation of RSV infection, ranging from asymptomatic illness to respiratory failure and death.[27] Most people who are symptomatic will experience an incubation period of about 4 to 7 days between exposure and development of symptoms.[25,27] The clinical presentation of RSV infection varies based on age and immune status. Infants and young children infected with RSV most commonly present with cold-like symptoms, including rhinorrhea, cough, sneezing, decrease in appetite, fever, and wheezing.[25] In adults infected with RSV, symptoms are usually mild or absent. If symptoms develop, these may include rhinorrhea, pharyngitis, cough, headache, fatigue, and fever.[25] Table 10–5 lists patient characteristics that increase the risk of developing severe disease due to RSV infection. Patients with severe disease, including pneumonia and bronchiolitis, may require hospitalization.[25,27] Symptoms that may accompany severe disease include difficulty breathing, dehydration, and acute respiratory distress.[25,27] Patients presenting with symptoms suggestive of severe disease should be referred to emergency medical care or a PCP immediately. Acute complications that may occur because of RSV infection include exacerbations of chronic obstructive pulmonary disease (COPD), asthma, and congestive heart failure (CHF) in older adults, and otitis media, hepatitis, and apnea in infants.[27] In addition, infection with RSV may be associated with chronic respiratory issues that persist once the infection resolves.[27]

Table 10–5. Characteristics associated with increased risk of severe disease with RSV[25]

Children
Premature infants
Age ≤6 months
Age <2 years with chronic lung disease or congenital heart disease
Immunocompromised
Neuromuscular disorders (including those associated with difficulty swallowing or clearing secretions)
Adults
Age ≥65 years
Chronic pulmonary or cardiovascular disease
Immunocompromised

Diagnosis

As clinical symptoms overlap with other respiratory viruses and bacteria, laboratory testing is required to confirm a diagnosis of RSV infection. Since infection with RSV is typically mild and self-limiting, diagnostic testing may not be necessary in all cases. The American Academy of Pediatrics recommends against routine virologic testing in children as a confirmed diagnosis of RSV infection does not change management practices in many cases.[28] It may be beneficial to perform testing for RSV in certain scenarios as listed in Box 10–1.

> **Box 10–1. Scenarios which may support RSV diagnostic testing**[25,26,29]
>
> - Patients at risk for severe disease (as described in Table 5)
> - Patients presenting with severe symptoms and/or symptoms that would require treatment
> - To inform cohorting/isolation to prevent transmission to high-risk patients or in hospital settings
> - To limit unnecessary additional diagnostic testing or antibiotic prescribing

The most commonly utilized tests include real-time reverse transcriptase-polymerase chain reaction (rRT-PCR) and antigen testing, and both upper and lower respiratory tract specimens may be sent for testing.[25] In infants and young children, both rRT-PCR and antigen testing may be effective in confirming the diagnosis, whereas only rRT-PCR testing is recommended in older children, adolescents, and adults due to decreased sensitivity and increased risk of false negative results with the use of antigen testing in this population.[25]

Physical Assessment

Patients should be evaluated for the presence of signs or symptoms consistent with RSV infection as discussed in the clinical presentation section. Patients most commonly present with mild, cold-like symptoms.[25] POCT for RSV requires collection of a nasopharyngeal swab specimen or a nasal aspirate or wash.[29]

Point-of-Care Testing

POCT for RSV most commonly utilizes rapid antigen testing and PCR technology.[30] Several tests are available to test for additional viruses in combination with RSV, including influenza and SARS-CoV-2, the causative virus of COVID-19 disease. In addition, at-home test kits are available for patient use. Examples of common POCTs for RSV are shown in Table 10–6 (this table does not include all POCTs available for RSV).

Table 10-6. Comparison of common POCTs available for RSV detection[30-32]

Target of test	Mechanism of testing	Example brands (time to result)	Comments
RSV alone	Rapid antigen	BD Veritor Plus System (10 minutes)	CLIA-waved test kit available for patients <6 years old
		BinaxNOW RSV Card (15 minutes)	For patients <5 years old
Combination RSV/Flu	Polymerase Chain Reaction (PCR)	cobas Influenza A/B & RSV (20 minutes)	Requires use with cobas Liat PCR System; no age restrictions
Combination RSV/Flu/ COVID-19	Polymerase Chain Reaction (PCR)	LabCorp Seasonal Respiratory Virus RT-PCR Test (Pixel by LabCorp) (1–2 days)	Available under FDA Emergency Use Authorization; Home collection kit for patients ≥2 years old; insurance accepted

Treatment

The treatment of RSV infection consists of supportive care alone for most patients.[33] Supportive care may include hydration, management of fever and pain with over-the-counter medications, supplemental oxygen (including mechanical ventilation if required), and control of secretions through suctioning of airways.[25,33] Most patients will be treated as outpatients and hospitalization is not commonly required.[25,27] Aerosolized ribavirin is the only FDA-approved medication currently available for the treatment of RSV in pediatric patients.[33] Due to high cost (average wholesale price reported as high as approximately $29,000 for one 6-gram vial), toxicities, questionable impact on clinical outcomes, and safety risk for health care professionals following exposure to aerosolized ribavirin, this medication is not used commonly in practice.[33,34] Instead, oral ribavirin may be considered for off-label use in patients with severe illness and/or those who are immunocompromised.[35] The goals of therapy for RSV infection include improvement in symptoms, faster resolution of disease, and potential for reduction in transmission to others by decreasing viral load.[33] In most immunocompetent people infected with RSV, resolution of infection typically occurs within 1 to 2 weeks.[25] There is a significant need for additional therapeutic options for management of RSV, especially for vulnerable patient populations that are at risk to progress to severe disease. Several antiviral agents are currently in development, including fusion inhibitors, which aim to prevent viral entry into the host cell, and replication inhibitors, which target viral replication or assembly.[33]

Indications for Referral

Figure 10-3. Algorithm for RSV POCT[25]

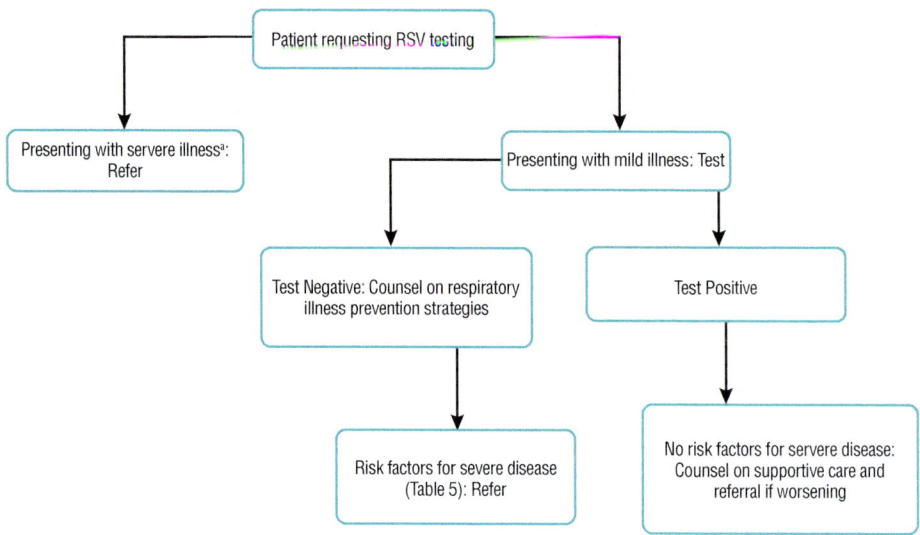

[a]Symptoms associated with severe illness include: shortness of breath, fever cyanosis, wheezing, worsening cough, dehydration, acute respiratory distress

Most patients do not require testing for RSV as this does not change management practices in most cases.[29] Box 10-1 lists certain clinical scenarios in which testing for RSV infection may be considered. Figure 10-3 provides a POCT algorithm that may be considered for RSV testing. Patients presenting with severe illness, including symptoms such as shortness of breath, fever, cyanosis, wheezing, worsening cough, dehydration, and/or acute respiratory distress, should be referred to emergency medical care or a PCP, as appropriate.[36] POCT may be considered in patients presenting with mild illness, such as cold-like symptoms. If a patient tests negative for RSV, the HCP may offer counseling on respiratory illness prevention strategies, including frequent hand washing, avoiding close contact with those who are infected, and cleaning frequently touched surfaces.[25] Patients who test positive for RSV and have risk factors for severe disease (Table 10-5) should be referred to a PCP, whereas patients without risk factors for severe disease and mild illness may receive counseling from an HCP on supportive care for management in the case of a positive test result, including hydration and use of over-the-counter medications for fever and pain control.[25,33] The HCP should also counsel patients who test positive to seek medical referral to a PCP if symptoms worsen and become consistent with severe illness (symptoms associated with severe illness are listed in Figure 10-3). In pediatric patients, additional worsening symptoms that indicate a need for referral include decreased activity, nasal flaring, bluish lips and fingernails, and poor intake of fluids.[36] There is a lack of clear guidance on the duration of time that patients infected with RSV should avoid contact with people who are at high risk of severe disease if transmission occurs. Most immunocompetent people with mild illness remain contagious for 3 to 8 days from symptom onset.[25] CDC guidelines for isolation precautions in health care settings suggest maintaining contact precautions (including standard precautions and masking) for the duration of symptomatic illness in those with RSV in the institutional setting.[37] Therefore, it would be reasonable to recommend that immunocompetent patients (excluding young infants) who test positive for RSV should avoid contact with high-risk patient populations for at least 8 days and for the duration of symptomatic illness, whichever is longer, if this is possible.[25,37]

Hepatitis C Virus Infection

HCV infection is a major cause of liver-related morbidity and mortality. HCV is transmitted by blood-to-blood contact, and individuals who are at the highest risk of infection include persons who use injection drugs, persons who received a blood transfusion prior to 1992, health care workers who are at risk for needle stick injuries, and children born to persons with HCV infection.[38] More than 4,000 new cases of HCV are reported each year in the United States.[38] However, due to under-reporting, it is estimated that more than 57,000 new cases occur each year in the United States.[38] About 2.4 million people are estimated to be living with HCV in the United States.[38] Over 15,000 yearly death certificates include HCV as a cause of death. Due to underdiagnosing, the actual number of deaths is likely higher.[38]

Clinical Presentation

HCV can cause both an acute infection (duration of infection less than 6 months) and a chronic infection (infection lasting longer than 6 months).[38] Some individuals will spontaneously clear the infection and subsequently do not progress to chronic infection, but more than half of those infected will develop chronic infection.[38] Of every 100 people infected with HCV, 5 to 25 individuals will develop cirrhosis within two decades.[38] Most patients with acute HCV are asymptomatic; however, the most common symptoms include fever, fatigue, dark urine, clay-colored stool, abdominal pain, loss of appetite, nausea, vomiting, joint pain, and jaundice.[38] Most individuals with chronic HCV also are asymptomatic unless the associated liver damage progresses to cirrhosis.[38] Complications of cirrhosis include hepatocellular carcinoma and decompensated liver disease, which can include esophageal varices, ascites, and hepatic encephalopathy.[38] Some individuals with chronic HCV develop symptoms that occur outside the liver, such as diabetes, glomerulonephritis, essential mixed cryoglobulinemia, porphyria cutanea tarda, and non-Hodgkin's lymphoma.[38]

Diagnosis

The CDC recommends that all adults be tested for HCV at least once in their lifetime, and all pregnant persons should be tested each pregnancy.[38] Individuals with ongoing risk of transmission should be tested on a routine basis.[38] The primary screening test is an HCV antibody test (anti-HCV).[38] If the antibody test is reactive, then a test for HCV RNA should be performed to confirm current infection.[38] See Table 10–7 below for criteria for interpretation of HCV tests.

Table 10–7. Interpretation of HCV test results

Test result	Interpretation
Anti-HCV non-reactive	Patient not infected or exposed
Anti-HCV reactive HCV RNA detected	Current HCV infection
Anti-HCV reactive HCV RNA not detected	No current HCV infection

Physical Assessment

Most patients with HCV are asymptomatic, so no signs or symptoms may be present that would be observed in a physical exam.[38] All currently approved POCTs require a finger stick blood sample to be drawn.[39]

Point-of-Care Testing

All currently available POCTs for HCV work by detecting the HCV antibody.[39] Example brands include Everlywell and iDNA, which are similar in cost.[38] Each POCT requires a finger stick blood sample that is sent to a lab, and results are available within one week.[39] As the CDC recommends testing all adults at least once in their lifetime for HCV, all adults qualify for POCT.[38] POCTs for HCV RNA are under development.

Treatment

All patients diagnosed with HCV qualify for treatment except those with a short life expectancy due to a non-HCV-related reason.[40] The goals of treatment are to reduce HCV-related morbidity and mortality, which includes halting the progression to end-stage liver disease and hepatocellular carcinoma.[40] The measurable treatment goal is sustained virologic response (SVR), which is confirmed by an undetectable HCV viral load at least 12 weeks after treatment ends.[40] Most patients can be treated with 8 to 12 weeks of oral direct-acting antiviral (DAA) treatment. Options for patients with any HCV genotype include sofosbuvir/velpatasvir and glecaprevir/pibrentasvir.[40] Options for patients with genotypes 1, 4, 5, or 6 include sofosbuvir/ledipasvir and elbasvir/grazoprevir. The choice of DAA regimen is likely driven by insurance coverage and other patient characteristics (e.g., comorbidities, potential drug–drug interactions, etc.). Further guidance is available for treatment of patients who were previously treated with a DAA regimen, have decompensated cirrhosis, are post-liver transplant, and/or have other unique characteristics.[40] Monitoring of DAA treatment is performed through laboratory testing. Counseling points for patients with HCV include avoiding alcohol, because alcohol can accelerate liver damage, as well as consuming a healthy diet and remaining physically active.[40] Counseling about the risk of transmission to others is also important.[40] See Figure Figure 10-4 below.

Figure 10–4. HCV POCT management algorithm

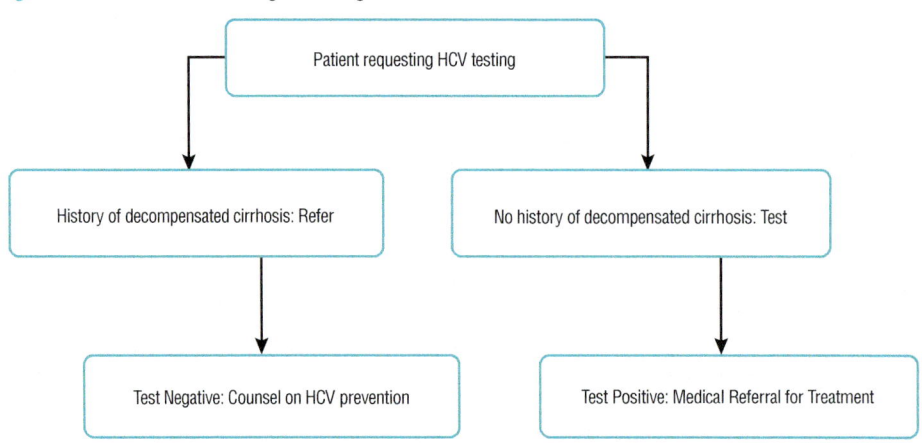

Indications for Referral

All patients who are diagnosed with HCV should be referred for medical treatment. Patients with signs/symptoms of decompensated cirrhosis (ascites, hepatic encephalopathy, variceal hemorrhage) should be referred for management and possible evaluation for liver transplant.[40]

Patient Cases

Patient Case 10–1 SOAP Note

Collect	Chief complaint
Subjective	"I need to find out if RSV is causing my symptoms."
	History of present illness (HPI)
	Patient AP is a 38-year-old woman who presents to the community pharmacy requesting testing for RSV. She works at a bank and reports that several of her colleagues have been out sick lately, and one of her colleagues reported testing positive for RSV. AP reports rhinorrhea, pharyngitis, headache, and fatigue, which have been present for the past 2 days. She is planning to travel to meet her niece for the first time this weekend (infant is 2 months old and was born premature), and she would like to confirm whether she is infected with RSV to determine if it is safe to be in contact with her niece.
Objective	Past medical history (PMH): hypothyroidism, seasonal allergies
	Family history (FH): non-contributory
	Social history (SH): married with no children, works at a bank, denies alcohol or illicit drug use
	Medication list: levothyroxine 100 mcg orally daily, loratadine 10 mg orally daily (only during allergy season in spring)
	Allergies: no known drug allergies (NKDA)
	Physical examination (PE):
	General appearance: 38-year-old woman in no acute distress, A&O x 3
	Vital signs (VS):
	BP: 118/70 mm Hg; pulse (P): 70 bpm; respiratory rate (RR): 18 breaths/minute; temperature: 97.9°F, height: 67 in; weight: 150 lbs (68 kg)
	Skin: warm, dry, and intact without rashes, lesions, or erythema; normal skin turgor
	Head, eyes, ears, nose, and throat (HEENT): Pupils are equal, round, and reactive to light and accommodation (PERRLA). Normal except for erythematous nasal mucosa associated with rhinorrhea and erythematous and swollen pharynx.
	Neck/lymph nodes: Neck is supple and there is no lymphadenopathy.
	Lungs/Thorax: Chest wall is symmetric and without deformity. No respiratory distress apparent. Lungs are clear to auscultation with no wheezing, rhonchi, or rales.
	Abdomen: Non-tender and non-distended.
	Review of symptoms (ROS) (only pertinent positives included):
	Constitutional symptoms: positive for fatigue

Patient Case 10-1 SOAP Note cont'd

	HEENT: positive for rhinorrhea and sore throat Neurological: positive for headache POCT results: RSV PCR testing (nasopharyngeal swab sample): positive
Assess	The patient's symptoms are consistent with mild RSV infection.[25] The patient does not have any symptoms consistent with severe infection, such as shortness of breath, signs of dehydration (as evidenced by normal skin turgor and general well appearance) or fever. RSV infection is confirmed with a positive PCR test result. Based on the history provided, the patient is immunocompetent and does not have risk factors for development of severe disease.[25] Goals for management of the patient's RSV infection include improvement in symptoms (including rhinorrhea, pharyngitis, headache, fatigue) and resolution of disease. The patient also mentioned that she is planning a visit to see her niece who was born prematurely 2 months ago. The patient's niece is at risk for severe disease if infected with RSV given age ≤6 months and history of prematurity.[25]
Plan	Following the POCT algorithm in Figure 3, the patient does not require referral to her PCP given mild disease and no risk factors for progression to severe disease. The HCP should provide information on supportive care for management of infection, including ensuring adequate hydration and using over-the-counter medications (such as acetaminophen) for pain or fever as needed. The HCP should counsel the patient on the typical duration of illness with RSV (1–2 weeks), inform the patient of signs/symptoms associated with severe disease, and recommend referral to a PCP or emergency medical care as appropriate, if these occur.[25] In addition, the HCP should recommend that the patient avoid contact with her niece if possible, because infection with RSV could lead to severe disease in her niece.
Implement	The HCP should confirm that the patient understands the plan for symptomatic management and referral, if needed, as discussed in the plan step. In addition, strategies for prevention of RSV infection may be discussed with the patient (i.e., hand washing, avoiding close contact with those who are infected, and cleaning frequently touched surfaces).[25] The HCP may recommend that the patient avoid contact with her high-risk niece for a minimum of 8 days following infection, or until symptoms resolve, whichever is longer.[25,37]
Monitor/ Follow-up	Clinical endpoints to be monitored include resolution of symptoms (rhinorrhea, pharyngitis, headache, and fatigue) and monitoring to ensure that symptoms do not progress. The patient should be informed of methods for PCP referral if symptoms do not improve or worsen. In addition, the HCP should confirm that the patient has a PCP available if referral is necessary.

Patient Case 10–2 SOAP Note

Collect	Chief complaint
Subjective	"My kid said I should be tested for hepatitis C, and I saw your flyer that you do those tests here now."
	HPI
	Patient KA is a 52-year-old man who comes to the pharmacy seeking a hepatitis C test. His daughter, who is in nursing school, learned that everyone should be screened for hepatitis C, so she suggested that he get a test. KA has no complaints except some swelling in his abdomen that his daughter thinks could be ascites, which has been present for several months. He admits to missing his yearly check-up with his HCP last week, and he hasn't rescheduled that appointment.
	PMH: hypertension for 5 years (controlled)
Objective	FH: Parents died of "natural causes" in their late 70s; two brothers alive with hypertension and obesity.
	SH: Drinks four cans of beer per night during the evening news for more than 30 years. Denies smoking and illicit drug use except for one time using IV drugs "a long time ago." Married for 25 years with two adult children.
	Medications: hydrochlorothiazide 25 mg orally daily Allergies: NKDA
	PE: General appearance: 52-year-old man in no acute distress, A&O x 3 VS: BP: 128/77 mm Hg; P: 81 bpm; RR: 18 breaths/minute; temperature: 98.7°F; height: 72 in; weight: 268 lbs (122 kg) Skin: intact, without rashes, lesions, or erythema HEENT: PERRLA, anicteric sclera, moist mucous membranes Abdomen: non-tender and distended
	ROS: The patient says that the swelling in his abdomen is symmetrical and throughout his belly area. He says it is uncomfortable and tight but is not painful. He denies any swelling in any other area of the body. The swelling started a few months ago, and he has noticed some increase in weight as his abdomen swelled. He has not tried anything to improve it and has not found anything that makes it worse. He denies any changes to his medications, allergies, or medical conditions besides those already listed.
	Laboratory test results: None available at time of patient encounter.
Assess	The patient is requesting an HCV test, but he also has concerning signs and symptoms of abdominal distension. The potential causes of abdominal distension are numerous and include malignancy, bowel obstruction, irritable bowel syndrome, and ascites. In this patient with risk factors for cirrhosis (chronic alcohol ingestion and prior IV drug use), ascites is a likely cause. Symmetrical, non-painful abdominal distension is also consistent with ascites. The patient does not have any other findings from the physical examination consistent with ascites or other cirrhosis complications.
	The goals of therapy for this patient would be to relieve the discomfort from the abdominal distension, identify the cause of the abdominal distension, and eliminate the cause if possible.

Patient Case 10-2 SOAP Note cont'd

Plan	Options at this point are to proceed with the HCV POCT or to recommend medical referral. While the HCV POCT would help determine if HCV is contributing to the abdominal distension, a more thorough medical work-up is likely needed to achieve the therapeutic goals.
	Therefore, the plan for this patient is:
	• Recommend medical referral ASAP to further evaluate abdominal distension.
	• Educate patient about some of the causes of abdominal distension, including liver-related causes, and the importance of a more in-depth evaluation to determine and try to eliminate the cause of his symptoms.
Implement	Offer to call patient's HCP to try to expedite the referral process.
Monitor/ Follow-up	Offer to follow-up with the patient and HCP to provide continuity of care and additional testing, vaccination, and medication-related services as appropriate after a diagnosis is made.

References

1. Chey WD, Leontiadis GI, Howden CW, Moss SF. ACG Clinical Guideline: Treatment of Helicobacter pylori Infection. *Am J Gastroenterol.* 2017;112(2):212–239. doi:10.1038/ajg.2016.563. Epub 2017 Jan 10. Erratum in: *Am J Gastroenterol.* 2018;113(7):1102.

2. Roberts LT, Issa PP, Sinnathamby ES, et al. Helicobacter Pylori: A Review of Current Treatment Options in Clinical Practice. *Life.* 2022;12(12):2038. doi:10.3390/life12122038

3. Connor BA. Helicobacter pylori. In: CDC Yellow Book 2020: Health Information for International Travel. Centers for Disease Control and Prevention. New York: Oxford University Press; 2017. Available at: https://wwwnc.cdc.gov/travel/yellowbook/2020/travel-related-infectious-diseases/helicobacter-pylori. Accessed August 9, 2024.

4. Fashner J, Gitu AC. Diagnosis and Treatment of Peptic Ulcer Disease and H. pylori Infection. *Am Fam Physician.* 2015;91(4):236–42.

5. Crowe SE. *Helicobacter pylori* Infection. *New England Journal of Medicine.* 2019;380:1158–65. doi:10.1056/NEJMcp1710945

6. Poly stat® *H. pylori* test [package insert]. Cortlandt Manor, NY: Polymedco, Inc.; 2014.

7. Accutest® *H. pylori* test [package insert]. Encino, CA: Jant Pharmacal Corporation; 2011.

8. Pharmacy Times. Wick JY. Nonprescription Self-Management of Functional Dyspepsia. Available at https://www.pharmacytimes.com/view/nonprescription-self-management-of-functional-dyspepsia. Accessed April 23, 2023.

9. Fernandez JM, Coyle EA. Chapter 139: Urinary Tract Infections. In: DiPiro JT, Yee GC, Haines ST, Nolin TD, Ellingrod VL, Posey L. eds. *DiPiro's Pharmacotherapy: Pathophysiologic Approach*, 12e. McGraw Hill; 2023. Accessed April 12, 2023.

10. Gupta K, Hooton TM, Naber KG, Wullt B, Colgan R, Miller LG, Moran GJ, Nicolle LE, Raz R, Schaeffer AJ, Soper DE; Infectious Diseases Society of America; European Society for Microbiology and Infectious Diseases. International clinical practice guidelines for the treatment of acute uncomplicated cystitis and pyelonephritis in women: A 2010 update by the Infectious Diseases Society of America and the European Society for Microbiology and Infectious Diseases. *Clin Infect Dis.* 2011;52(5):e103–20. doi:10.1093/cid/ciq257

11. Santos M, Mariz M, Tiago I, Martins J, Alarico S, Ferreira P. A review on urinary tract infections diagnostic methods: Laboratory-based and point-of-care approaches. *J Pharm Biomed Anal.* 2022;219:114889. doi:10.1016/j.jpba.2022.114889

12. Nicolle LE, Gupta K, Bradley SF, Colgan R, DeMuri GP, Drekonja D, Eckert LO, Geerlings SE, Köves B, Hooton TM, Juthani-Mehta M, Knight SL, Saint S, Schaeffer AJ, Trautner B, Wullt B, Siemieniuk R. Clinical Practice Guideline for the Management of Asymptomatic Bacteriuria: 2019 Update by the Infectious Diseases Society of America. *Clin Infect Dis.* 2019;68(10):e83–e110. doi:10.1093/cid/ciy1121

13. Wagenlehner FME, Bjerklund Johansen TE, Cai T, et al. Epidemiology, definition and treatment of complicated urinary tract infections. *Nature Reviews Urology.* 2020;17(10):586–600. doi:10.1038/s41585-020-0362-4

14. Schulz L, Hoffman RJ, Pothof J, et al. Top Ten Myths Regarding the Diagnosis and Treatment of Urinary Tract Infections. *J Emerg Med.* 2016;51(1):25–30. doi:10.1016/j.jemermed.2016.02.009

15. Queremel Milani DA, Jialal I. Urinalysis. In: StatPearls[Internet]. StatPearls Publishing: Treasure Island (FL); 2023. Accessed April 16, 2023. https://www.ncbi.nlm.nih.gov/books/NBK557685/.

16. Beahm NP, Nicolle LE, Bursey A, Smyth DJ, Tsuyuki RT. The assessment and management of urinary tract infections in adults: Guidelines for pharmacists. *Can Pharm J (Ott)*. 2017;150(5):298–305. doi:10.1177/1715163517723036

17. Simerville JA, Maxted WC, Pahira JJ. Urinalysis: a comprehensive review [published correction appears in Am Fam Physician. 2006 Oct 1;74(7):1096]. *Am Fam Physician*. 2005;71(6): 1153–1162.

18. Testing.com. The 3 Best At-Home UTI Tests of 2022. Available at https://www.testing.com/tests/at-home-uti-test/. Accessed April 23, 2023.

19. AZO® Test Strips [package insert]. Cromwell, CT: I-Health, Inc.; 2012.

20. Uristat® Relief PAKTM [package insert]. Langhorne, PA: INSIGHT Pharmaceuticals, LLC.; 2011.

21. Little P, Merriman R, Turner S, et al. Presentation, pattern, and natural course of severe symptoms, and role of antibiotics and antibiotic resistance among patients presenting with suspected uncomplicated urinary tract infection in primary care: observational study. *BMJ*. 2010;340:b5633. doi:10.1136/bmj.b5633

22. Page A, Owen JA, Goode JR, et al. Pharmacist-initiated treatment of minor conditions: A call to action. *J Am Pharm Assoc*. 2021;61(1):13–19. doi:10.1016/j.japh.2020.09.021

23. National Alliance of State Pharmacy Associations. Pharmacist Prescribing: "Test and Treat." Richmond, VA: NASPA. Available at: https://naspa.us/resource/pharmacist-prescribing-for-strep-and-flu-test-and-treat/. Accessed April 18, 2023.

24. Beahm NP, Smyth DJ, Tsuyuki RT. Outcomes of Urinary Tract Infection Management by Pharmacists (RxOUTMAP): A study of pharmacist prescribing and care in patients with uncomplicated urinary tract infections in the community. *Can Pharm J (Ott)*. 2018;151(5):305–314. doi:10.1177/1715163518781175

25. Centers for Disease Control and Prevention. Respiratory Syncytial Virus Infection (RSV). Atlanta, GA: CDC. Available at: https://www.cdc.gov/rsv/index.html. Accessed March 28, 2023.

26. Barr R, Green CA, Sande CJ, et al. Respiratory syncytial virus: Diagnosis, prevention and management. *Ther Adv Infectious Dis*. 2019;6:1–9. doi:10.1177/2049936119865798

27. Kaler J, Hussain A, Patel K, et al. Respiratory Syncytial Virus: A Comprehensive Review of Transmission, Pathophysiology, and Manifestation. Cureus. 2023;15(3):e36342. doi:10.7759/cureus. 36342

28. Ralston SL, Lieberthal AS, Meissner HC, et al. American Academy of Pediatrics. Clinical Practice Guideline: The Diagnosis, Management, and Prevention of Bronchiolitis. Pediatrics. 2014; 134(5):e1475–e1502. doi:10.1542/peds. 2014-2742

29. Drysdale SB, Kelly DF. How to use…respiratory viral studies. *Arch Dis Child Educ Pract Ed*. 2019; 104(5):274–278. doi:10.1136/archdischild-2016-311858

30. Bernstein DI, Mejias A, Rath B, Woods CW, Deeter JP. Summarizing Study Characteristics and Diagnostic Performance of Commercially Available Tests for Respiratory Syncytial Virus: A Scoping Literature Review in the COVID-19 Era. *J Appl Lab Med*. 2023;8(2):353–371. doi:10.1093/jalm/jfac058

31. cobas® Influenza A/B & RSV [package insert]. Branchburg, NJ: Roche Molecular Systems, Inc.; 2018.

32. Labcorp® Seasonal Respiratory Virus RT-PCR Test [package insert]. Burlington, NC: Laboratory Corporation of America; 2022.

33. Domachowske JB, Anderson EJ, Goldstein M. The Future of Respiratory Syncytial Virus Disease Prevention and Treatment. *Infect Dis Ther*. 2021; 10(Suppl 1):47–60. doi:10.1007/s40121-020-00383-6

34. UpToDate, Inc. UpToDate drug monograph - ribavirin (oral inhalation). Available at: https://www.uptodate.com. Accessed April 11, 2023.

35. Nam HH, Ison MG. Respiratory syncytial virus infection in adults. BMJ. 2019;366:l5021. doi:10.1136/bmj.l5021

36. American Lung Association. Respiratory Syncytial Virus. Available at: https://www.lung.org/lung-health-diseases/lung-disease-lookup/rsv/rsv-in-adults. Accessed April 12, 2023.

37. Centers for Disease Control and Prevention. Siegel JD, Rhinehart E, Jackson M, et al. 2007 Guideline for Isolation Precautions: Preventing Transmission of Infectious Agents in Healthcare Settings. Atlanta, GA: CDC. Available at: http://www.cdc.gov/infectioncontrol/guidelines/isolation/index.html. Accessed April 12, 2023.

38. Centers for Disease Control and Prevention. Hepatitis C. Atlanta, GA: CDC. Available at: https://www.cdc.gov/hepatitis/hcv/index.htm. Accessed April 9, 2023.

39. Testing.com. At-Home Hepatitis C Test. Available at https://www.testing.com/tests/at-home-hepatitis-c-test/. Accessed April 9, 2023.

40. American Association for the Study of Liver Diseases–Infectious Diseases Society of America. HCV Guidance: Recommendations for testing, managing, and treating hepatitis C. Alexandria, VA: AASLD-IDSA. Available at http://www.hcvguidelines.org. Accessed April 9, 2023.

CHAPTER 11

Diabetes

Clark Kebodeaux, PharmD, BCACP

Key Points

- Diabetes is a significant cause of U.S. health care spending and the 8th leading cause of death in the United States.
- The use of point-of-care testing (POCT) to identify and refer patients with prediabetes can delay progression to type 2 diabetes.
- HCPs should be familiar with glycemic levels indicating prediabetes and diagnosis of type 2 diabetes to ensure appropriate referral after POCT.
- Lifestyle changes, including physical activity and nutrition, supported by appropriate screening and monitoring can reduce morbidity and mortality related to diabetes.
- Referring patients to a DPP with a focus on weight reduction through caloric restriction and increased physical activity can impact progression to type 2 diabetes.

The impact of diabetes morbidity and mortality is high, and the condition is a significant public health priority. In 2021, diabetes was the 8th leading cause of death (31.1 deaths per 100,000) in the United States (U.S.), where it was responsible for over 103,000 deaths.[1] Diabetes has a substantial individual burden; more than 38 million visits to PCPs occur annually in which the primary diagnosis is type 2 diabetes.[2] It is estimated that diabetes is responsible for $237 billion dollars in direct health care costs to the U.S., in addition to $90 billion in indirect costs due to death, disability, and reduced productivity.[3] Individuals with diabetes are likely to spend 2 to 3 times as much on their health care as those not diagnosed with the disease.[3]

Over the last two decades, the annual rate of diabetes diagnosis has increased continually in the U.S. The prevalence of diabetes in the U.S. from 2017–2020 was estimated to be 14.7% of the adult population 18 years or older.[4] This population included more than 37 million adults, among which 8.5 million individuals did not report a diagnosis of diabetes and were unaware that their glycemic level reached the criteria for diagnosis. In contrast, the estimated prevalence of diabetes in adults in the U.S. was 10.3% from 2001–2004.[4] In 2019, the incidence of diabetes in U.S. adults was 5.9 per 1000 people, resulting in 1.4 million new cases of diagnosed diabetes.[5] The prevalence of diabetes increases with age (29.2% in adults over 65 years old) and is strongly correlated with obesity; 89.9% of U.S. adults diagnosed with diabetes have a BMI greater than 25 kg/m2.[4,5] Geographic rates of obesity and physical inactivity are similar to rates of diagnosed diabetes.[5] Given the constantly increasing prevalence of diabetes and the relatively large population with undiagnosed diabetes in the United States, POCT and treatment are important components of strategies to reduce morbidity and mortality by identifying patients with diabetes and helping them improve their glycemic control.

Clinical Presentation

Diabetes most commonly presents as hyperglycemia with polyuria and polydipsia. Other symptoms of diabetes include weight loss, fatigue, vision changes, neuropathy, and reduced immune function.[6] While patients may be diagnosed without symptoms of hyperglycemia, some patients present with diabetic ketoacidosis (DKA)—a serious and potentially life-threatening hyperglycemic illness that requires acute assessment and treatment. Fifty percent of children diagnosed with type 1 diabetes present with DKA.[7] Symptoms may vary based on the specific diagnosis of diabetes as described below.

The complications of uncontrolled hyperglycemia are significant. In the absence of appropriate testing and treatment, an elevated glucose burden can result in serious microvascular problems, including nerve damage, vision/hearing loss, and poor oral and foot health. Specifically, patients diagnosed with diabetes have higher risk for cardiovascular disease, chronic kidney disease (CKD), and mental health diagnoses.[8]

Diagnosis

The American Diabetes Association (ADA) classifies diabetes in the following manner:[7]

- Type 1 diabetes
- Type 2 diabetes
- Gestational diabetes mellitus
- Diabetes secondary to a known cause

Type 1 diabetes is a result of autoimmune-mediated destruction of beta-cells in the pancreas.[7] While not exclusive to children, onset and diagnosis of type 1 diabetes typically occur early in life. Type 2 diabetes is the most prevalent form (this chapter will focus primarily on type 2 diabetes); more than 90% of diagnosed patients have type 2 diabetes. Gestational diabetes mellitus (GDM) is diabetes that presents during pregnancy; however, it may also represent preexisting diabetes that was detected as part of routine pregnancy screening. Diabetes secondary to a known cause could include drug-induced diabetes, diabetes due to diseases of the pancreas, or other monogenic types of diabetes.[7] Early identification, treatment, and prevention of mild hyperglycemia can prevent the patient from progressing to a diagnosis of type 2 diabetes. This initial level of glucose intolerance is referred to as 'prediabetes'.

The ADA and the American Association of Clinical Endocrinology (AACE) are the primary resources used by health care professionals in the United States to define diagnosis of diabetes. In their definitions of prediabetes, ADA and AACE agree that impaired fasting glucose (IFG) is indicated by a fasting plasma glucose (FPG) level of 100 mg/dL to 125 mg/dL, whereas impaired glucose tolerance (IGT) is indicated by a plasma glucose (PG) level of 140 to 199 mg/dL 2 hours after an oral glucose tolerance test (OGTT) or a hemoglobin A1C level between 5.7% and 6.4%.[7,9] These values are critical knowledge for HCPs conducting POCT, as identifying prediabetes can help patients identify pharmacologic and nonpharmacologic treatments or lifestyle changes to reduce their individual risk.

ADA and AACE agree on the following criteria for diagnosis of type 2 diabetes:[7,9]

- FPG ≥126 mg/dL (no food for 8 hours prior to test)
- 2-h PG ≥200 mg/dL after OGTT
- A1C ≥6.5%
- Random PG ≥200 mg/dL

A1C remains the gold standard for diagnosis and AACE recommended A1C as a screening tool for prediabetes.[9] Most POCT tests described below will require repeat or confirmatory testing to establish a definitive diagnosis of diabetes.

Physical Assessment

HCPs conducting POCT for diabetes must be familiar with glucose meters and appropriate lancing technique to ensure accurate results. Other physical assessment techniques may be performed to assess diabetes-related comorbidities, including cardiovascular disease or obesity, but these are not essential for appropriate sample collection via fingerstick for diabetes testing. Any patient who has been diagnosed with diabetes will require chronic care with appropriate physical assessment at diagnosis and should be monitored for complications.

Point-of-Care Testing

POCT devices for diabetes serve multiple purposes for HCPs and patients. Blood glucose meters are the primary choice for initial screening and monitoring the progression of the disease. ADA states that "people with diabetes should be provided with blood glucose monitoring devices as indicated by their circumstances, preferences, and treatment," and recent technological advances allow continuous glucose monitoring (CGM) for patients already diagnosed with type 2 diabetes.[10] While current CGM devices do not allow for POCT, CGM will likely surpass home blood glucose monitoring (BGM) as the primary monitoring method as the technology becomes more ubiquitous. BGM should be a critical part of any individualized diabetes plan when appropriate, and HCPs should be prepared to educate patients on BGM and utilize blood glucose meter devices for POCT testing when appropriate.

POCT screening tools for diabetes measure PG or A1C. Most meters are designed to measure PG, but CLIA-waived A1C kits are available for health care professionals and patients. Note that many CLIA-waived analyzers may also be available to measure PG or A1C as part of multiple screening assays or other laboratory tests. A summary of different types of available POCTs is included in Table 11–1.

Table 11-1. Sample of available POCTs for diabetes[11,12,21-24]

Example brands A1C testing	Blood sample size (microliters)	Cost comparison	Key points
A1CNow	0.5	$$	• Commercial facing A1C test • Should not be used for diagnosis
Blood glucose meters[a]			
Abbott FreeStyle Lite	0.3	$$	• Small blood sample size needed
CareSens N Voice	0.5	$$$	• Voice/audio in English and Spanish for patients with visual impairments
Countour Next One	0.6	$$$	• Bluetooth • smartLIGHT backlight for target ranges
EasyMax NG	0.6	$	• Large display • No coding

[a]Not a conclusive list

POCT A1C tests allow patients and HCPs to quickly assess results in under 5 minutes. This device uses a diluted blood sample to conjugate blue microparticles to anti-A1C antibodies using a reagent strip.[11] The total amount of microparticles is used to estimate the glycosylated hemoglobin and provide an A1C result. Note that this device should not be used for diagnostic purposes, but it can provide an A1C result for screening purposes.[11]

Many different meters are available to help patients and HCPs perform BGM. Each meter utilizes a test strip that measures the amount of glucose in a small blood sample by interacting with glucose oxidase or glucose dehydrogenase; this enzymatic interaction produces a small amount of electric current that is measured and converted to a glucose reading.[7,12]

In September 2020, FDA published a Final Guidance document entitled 'Blood Glucose Monitoring Test Systems for Prescription Point-of-Care Use' alongside a second guidance document intended to address BGM for home use.[13] For the first time, FDA distinguished BGM devices intended for POCT professional health care settings from BGM devices intended for home use for self-monitoring by patients. Specifically, this guidance was intended to ensure accuracy and safety by distinguishing testing in acute settings or long-term care facilities from testing by healthy users measuring PG at home. As a part of FDA's approach to regulating blood glucose meters for home use, all meters approved by FDA and sold over-the-counter (OTC) were automatically CLIA-waived. In addition, manufacturers supplied data to help ensure implementation of appropriate cleaning and disinfection procedures, as well as additional studies needed to support the requirements of testing in professional settings. While all BGM devices will remain CLIA-waived, these devices will contain labeling that includes the statements "Rx Only" and "can only be sold to health care professionals."[13]

POCT devices for diabetes for either home or professional use should function for all adults who would benefit from screening or use the device for chronic management of diabetes; however, several factors affect the accuracy of such devices under different circumstances.[10] Diabetes testing devices must be stored and used at room temperature, and the enzymatic reaction can be affected by temperature, humidity, and altitude. Most devices contain error messages that should prevent inaccurate results from being presented. The manufacturer's instructions for POCT devices should always be followed. Some pharmacologic treatments can affect glucose readings, but such effects are typically small and within the range of acceptable error. Treatments that can affect glucose testing results include acetaminophen (may decrease readings), uncontrolled gout (uric acid decreases readings), ascorbic acid, and L-dopa (variable effects).[14]

Given the number of meters available in the marketplace, HCPs must be familiar with each manufacturer's instructions to ensure that POCTs are administered appropriately. While sample testing instructions are covered in a previous chapter, a few items specific to testing PG are important to remember[15]:

- Ensure that the patient is aware of any pre-test instructions (if a fasting reading is preferred) or a full dietary history is taken to help interpret the PG result.
- Fingerstick devices should be used only once and properly disposed; avoid lancing devices that have not been approved for multiple patients.
- Per FDA regulations above, all blood glucose devices should be appropriately cleaned and sanitized between uses according to the manufacturer's instructions.

HCPs who plan to do POCT in long-term care facilities should ensure that fingerstick devices belonging to individual patients are appropriately labeled and not used for other patients to reduce the risk of spreading infectious agents such as hepatitis B virus (HBV).[15]

Treatment of Disease

Pharmacologic treatment for type 2 diabetes is chronic, complex and beyond the scope of this chapter. POCT testing plays a critical role in identifying prediabetes and undiagnosed diabetes, as well as helping diagnosed patients monitor and control glucose.

In screening and educating patients about the risks of diabetes, HCPs who perform POCT testing for diabetes can play a critical role in the prevention or delay of the progression to type 2 diabetes. For each POCT encounter, providers should be prepared to have a discussion regarding thresholds for diagnosis, blood glucose targets based on diagnosis, and the role of A1C in PG in monitoring disease progression. According to ADA, all patients can benefit from the following nonpharmacologic interventions to promote a healthy lifestyle[16]:

- Referral to a Diabetes Prevention Program (DPP),[17] with a focus on weight reduction through caloric restriction and increased physical activity
- Changes in eating patterns specific to patient-centered goals can impact prediabetes and progression to type 2 diabetes (nutrition)
- Engaging in 150 minutes of moderate to intense exercise every week has been shown to improve prediabetes (physical activity)

Some adult patients may benefit from pharmacologic interventions, such as metformin, if they have elevated BMI (≥ 35 kg/m^2), fasting blood glucose (FBG) ≥ 110 mg/dL, and A1C $\geq 6.0\%$.[16] All patients at risk for prediabetes after initial POCT results are obtained should be referred to an appropriate HCP for additional risk assessment and treatment based on individual needs.

Indications for Referral

The U.S. Preventive Services Task Force (USPSTF) recommends that "all nonpregnant adults aged 35 to 70 years seen in primary care settings who have overweight or obesity (defined as a BMI ≥25 and ≥30) and no symptoms of diabetes" should be screened for prediabetes via POCT or other standard laboratory assessment.[18] While any patient who meets the criteria for prediabetes or type 2 diabetes should be referred to an appropriate HCP, some patients will meet hypoglycemic or hyperglycemic thresholds that necessitate immediate referral to care. For example, patients who present with severe hyperglycemia such as PG >360 mg/dL should be screened for DKA and referred to emergent care for appropriate treatment.[7]

Hypoglycemia is typically defined as a PG reading of <70 mg/dL with symptoms such as sweating, shaking, general unwell feeling, confusion, hunger, and irritability. The clinical threshold for hypoglycemia is PG <70 mg/dL, and any patient meeting this criterion should be assessed for symptoms and hypoglycemia awareness. Patients who are conscious should receive 15 g of simple carbohydrates and should be tested again in 15 minutes to assess hypoglycemia. Patients who do not respond to treatment or patients who are initially symptomatic and have a reading of <54 mg/dL should be referred for emergent care and appropriate treatment.[19]

Patient Cases

Patient Case 11–1 SOAP Note

Collect **Subjective**	Chief complaint
	A 58-year-old man presents to a diabetes screening event at a local community center hosted annually to reach the local community. The patient presents with no symptoms, but he would like to be screened because his father was diagnosed with type 2 diabetes 20 years ago. The patient is the primary source of information at this event.
	History of Present Illness (HPI)
	Patient is seeking screening for type 2 diabetes pursuant to family history. Patient arrived at 0830 and intentionally fasted for more than 8 hours to ensure the most accurate reading. Patient is physically active and walks 2 days/week.
Objective	Past medical history (PMH): (+) hypertension
	Family history (FH): (+) first degree relative with type 2 diabetes
	Social history (SH): (-) tobacco, alcohol use
	Medication list: amlodipine 10 mg orally once daily, multiple vitamins infusion (MVI) orally once daily (OTC), vitamin B complex orally 1 daily (OTC)
	Allergies: no known drug allergies (NKDA)
	Physical examination (PE)/vital signs (VS): height: 70 in; weight: 212 lbs (self-reported)
	POCT results: FBG: 111 mg/dL
Assess	Patient took the Prediabetes Risk Test20 as part of the intake procedure prior to FBG screening (a score of 5 or higher indicates increased risk for prediabetes):
	1. Age 50–59 years (2 points) 2. Man (1 point) 3. Gestational diabetes (N/A) 4. Father with diabetes (1 point) 5. Diagnosed with HTN (1 point) 6. Physically active (0 points) 7. Weight category (2 points)
	Total Score = 7 points Patient's FBG reading was between 100 mg/dL and 125 mg/dL, indicating that he had increased risk of prediabetes.
Plan	Patient should be referred to his PCP for confirmatory testing and assessment of the patients' risk for prediabetes or type 2 diabetes. Patient was eligible for referral based on the results of POCT FBG. A second round of tests would be needed, including an A1C test, to assess individual risk.
Implement	In addition to referral to his PCP, the patient may benefit from enrolling in a Diabetes Prevention Program (DPP). Regardless of the confirmatory results, the patient would benefit from education, empowerment, and self-management related to changes in eating patterns to prevent progression to type 2 diabetes, as well as increasing physical activity to 150 minutes per week of moderate-intense exercise from (2 sessions/week).
Monitor/ Follow-up	After confirmatory results from his PCP, the patient should work toward a patient-centered goal of weight loss to reduce glycemic burden and the risk of progression to type 2 diabetes. The patient should follow up with his HCP based on the results of the test or attend DPP appointments based on successful enrollment in the program.

Patient Case 11–2 SOAP Note

Collect	Chief complaint/ HPI
Subjective	A 46-year-old woman presents to an outpatient clinic for a diabetes follow-up appointment. The patient was diagnosed with type 2 diabetes 6 years ago and has since improved her A1C control based on this diagnosis.
	After being checked in and moved to the assessment room, the patient reported a general feeling of weakness and blurry vision. The patient did not eat breakfast prior to the visit and left her blood glucose meter at home.
Objective	PMH: (+) type 2 diabetes, hypertension
	FH: (+) mother and father dx with type 2 diabetes
	SH: (+) tobacco, (-) alcohol use
	Medication list: lisinopril 20 mg orally once daily, metformin 1000 mg orally twice daily, empagliflozin 25 mg orally once daily, insulin glargine 12 U subcutaneously once daily in the morning
	Allergies: NKDA
	VS: BP: 116/82 mm Hg; pulse: 72 bpm; height: 64 in; weight, 163 lb
	Laboratory test results: A1C: 7.4%; eGFR: 84 mL/min/1.73 m^2
	POCT results: PG: 68 mg/dL
Assess	Patient is experiencing stage 1 hypoglycemia secondary to pharmacologic treatment of type 2 diabetes and fasting prior to scheduled follow-up. Patient's type 2 diabetes is currently uncontrolled per ADA/AACE A1C goal of 7%. Patient did not take her medications this morning without a morning meal to ensure an on-time arrival to clinic.
Plan	Assess the patient for symptoms and hypoglycemia awareness. If she is conscious, the patient should receive 15 g of simple carbohydrates and should be tested again in 15 minutes to assess hypoglycemia.
Implement	Patient received four glucose tablets after confirmatory symptoms consistent with hypoglycemia and a POCT result of 68 mg/dL. Patient noted resolution of symptoms, and a second POCT administered 15 minutes later obtained a level of 124 mg/dL.
Monitor/ Follow-up	While the patient responded to treatment, the patient should be educated about hypoglycemia awareness and the importance of self-monitoring and treatment. The patient's type 2 diabetes is treated with basal insulin, metformin, and an SGLT2 agent. Future adjustment of the patient's medications may be warranted based on a history of frequent hypoglycemic episodes.

References

1. Centers for Disease Control and Prevention. National Center for Health Statistics. Atlanta, GA: CDC. Available at: https://www.cdc.gov/nchs/fastats/diabetes.htm. Accessed March 20, 2023.

2. Santo L, Kang K. National Ambulatory Medical Care Survey: 2019 National Summary Tables. Available at: https://stacks.cdc.gov/view/cdc/123251. Accessed June 3, 2024.

3. American Diabetes Association. Economic Costs of Diabetes in the U.S. in 2017. *Diabetes Care.* 2018;41(5):917–928. doi:10.2337/dci18-0007

4. Centers for Disease Control and Prevention. National Diabetes Statistics Report. Atlanta, GA: CDC. Available at: https://www.cdc.gov/diabetes/data/statistics-report/index.html. Accessed March 20, 2023.

5. Centers for Disease Control and Prevention. National and State Diabetes Trends. Atlanta, GA: CDC. Available at: https://www.cdc.gov/diabetes/library/reports/reportcard/national-state-diabetes-trends.html. Accessed March 28, 2023.

6. ElSayed NA, Aleppo G, Aroda VR, et al. 2. Classification and Diagnosis of Diabetes: Standards of Care in Diabetes-2023 [published correction appears in Diabetes Care. 2023 Feb 01] [published correction appears in Diabetes Care. 2023 Sep 1;46(9):1715]. *Diabetes Care.* 2023;46(Suppl 1):S19–S40. doi:10.2337/dc23-S002

7. Centers for Disease Control and Prevention. Prevent Diabetes Complications. Atlanta, GA: CDC. Available at: https://www.cdc.gov/diabetes/managing/problems.html. Accessed March 30, 2023.

8. Blonde L, Umpierrez GE, Reddy SS, et al. American Association of Clinical Endocrinology Clinical Practice Guideline: Developing a Diabetes Mellitus Comprehensive Care Plan-2022 Update [published correction appears in Endocr Pract. 2023 Jan; 29(1):80–81]. *Endocr Pract.* 2022;28(10):923–1049. doi:10.1016/j.eprac.2022.08.002

9. ElSayed NA, Aleppo G, Aroda VR, et al. 7. Diabetes Technology: Standards of Care in Diabetes-2023. *Diabetes Care.* 2023;46(Suppl 1):S111–S127. doi:10.2337/dc23-S007

10. Polymer Technology Systems, Inc. A1CNow® [package insert]. Available at: https://ptsdiagnostics.com/wp-content/uploads/2018/08/pn_91076_rev._d_pkg_insert_a1cnow_en%EF%80%A2fr_ca__otc.pdf. Accessed April 16, 2023.

11. Abbott Diabetes Care Inc. Abbott® Freestyle Lite [package insert]. Available at: https://www.freestyle.abbott/ca-en/blood-glucose-meters/freestyle-lite.html. Accessed April 16, 2023.

12. U.S. Food and Drug Administration. Blood Glucose Monitoring Test Systems for Prescription Point-of-Care Use, September 2020. Silver Spring, MD: FDA. Available at: https://www.fda.gov/media/119829/download. Accessed April 16, 2023.

13. Ginsberg BH. Factors affecting blood glucose monitoring: Sources of errors in measurement. *J Diabetes Sci Technol.* 2009;3(4):903–913. doi:10.1177/193229680900300438

14. Centers for Disease Control and Prevention. Frequently Asked Questions (FAQs) regarding Assisted Blood Glucose Monitoring and Insulin Administration. Atlanta, GA: CDC. Available at: https://www.cdc.gov/injectionsafety/providers/blood-glucose-monitoring_faqs.html. Accessed April 16, 2023.

15. ElSayed NA, Aleppo G, Aroda VR, et al. 7. Diabetes Technology: Standards of Care in Diabetes–2023. Diabetes Care. 2023;46(Suppl 1):S111–S127. doi:10.2337/dc23-S007

16. Centers for Disease Control and Prevention. National Diabetes Prevention Program. Atlanta, GA: CDC. Available at: https://www.cdc.gov/diabetes/prevention/index.html. Accessed April 16, 2023.

17. U.S. Preventive Services Task Force, Davidson KW, Barry MJ, et al. Screening for Prediabetes and Type 2 Diabetes: U.S. Preventive Services Task Force Recommendation Statement. *JAMA.* 2021;326(8): 736–743. doi:10.1001/jama.2021.12531

18. ElSayed NA, Aleppo G, Aroda VR, et al. 6. Glycemic Targets: Standards of Care in Diabetes-2023. *Diabetes Care.* 2023;46(Suppl 1):S97–S110. doi:10.2337/dc23-S006

19. Centers for Disease Control and Prevention. Prediabetes Risk Test. Atlanta, GA: CDC. Available at: https://www.cdc.gov/diabetes/prevention/pdf/Prediabetes-Risk-Test-Final.pdf. Accessed April 16, 2023.

20. American Diabetes Association. Meters: Consumer Guide. Available at: https://consumerguide.diabetes.org/collections/meters. Accessed April 17, 2023.

21. i-SENS, Inc. CareSens® N Voice [package insert]. Available at: https://i-sens.com/pdf/en/2021/PGA1E3384-REV1-CS-N-Voice-N-ISO-M-Manual-CE-EN_CareSoft.pdf. Accessed April 17, 2023.

22. Ascensia Diabetes Care Holdings AG. Countour® Next One [User Guide]. Available at: https://www.ascensiadiabetes.com/siteassets/bgm-new/cno/cno-english-user-guide.pdf. Accessed April 17, 2023.

23. EPS Bio Technology Corp. EasyMax NG [User Guide]. Available at: https://www.oaktree-health.com/Manuals/EasyMax-NG-Manual.pdf. Accessed April 17, 2023.

CHAPTER 12

Dyslipidemia and Liver Function Abnormalities

Katelyn Johnson, PharmD, MS, BCACP and
Michael Hegener, PharmD, BCACP

Key Points

- The ACC/AHA Task Force on Clinical Practice Guidelines recommends that all adults aged 20 years and older complete screening for dyslipidemia every 4 to 6 years.
- The ASCVD Risk Estimator should be used in addition to a lipid panel to evaluate patients' risk of ASCVD and guide selection of pharmacotherapy.
- HCPs may perform lipid panel and liver transaminase monitoring via CLIA-waived POCT devices in their practice. Devices may vary by analytes measured, portability, storage requirements, and cost.
- Lowering LDL remains the primary target for pharmacotherapy. Statins are effective at lowering LDL and are typically well tolerated. HCPs may initiate and monitor statin therapy if permitted by state law.
- Patients presenting with liver or kidney disease, pregnancy, hypertriglyceridemia, or contraindications to statin therapy should be referred to their PCP.
- Routine periodic monitoring of transaminases in all patients on statin therapy is not recommended. AST and ALT should be assessed at baseline and then only if symptoms suggesting hepatoxicity develop.
- Patients with a persistent increase (remains elevated with repeat testing) in AST or ALT of >3 times the ULN should be referred to a PCP for further evaluation.

Dyslipidemia is a chronic condition in adults characterized by abnormal cholesterol values. Serum cholesterol is carried through the blood by lipoproteins and serves several important roles. Cholesterol aids in digestion and is necessary to form cell membranes and produce hormones and vitamins.[1] Abnormal cholesterol levels may have negative health effects and increase an individual's risk of atherosclerotic cardiovascular disease (ASCVD), which includes heart attack and stroke.[2] A lipid panel or profile may be ordered or conducted by HCPs to measure and calculate cholesterol levels. Test results are reported in milligrams per deciliter of blood (mg/dL) and include total cholesterol, low-density lipoprotein (LDL), high-density lipoprotein (HDL), and triglycerides.[1] Total cholesterol is a measure of LDL, HDL, and triglyceride levels. LDL or "bad" cholesterol can accumulate and contribute to fat buildup or plaques present in arteries, which may cause atherosclerosis, a condition that narrows or hardens arteries over time.[3,4] HDL or "good" cholesterol serves a protective role by transporting a portion of LDL from arteries, returning it to the liver where it undergoes degradation. Triglycerides are the most common type of fat in the body.[3]

High cholesterol, or hyperlipidemia, is a common condition in adults 20 years and older in the United States. Between 2017 and 2020, the prevalence of borderline high total cholesterol (≥200 mg/dL) and high total cholesterol (≥240 mg/dL) was 34.7% (86.4 million Americans) and 10.0% (24.7 million Americans), respectively. Non-Hispanic (NH) white, NH Asian, and Hispanic adults had a marginally higher prevalence of hyperlipidemia compared to NH Black adults, although the prevalence was similar. In the same survey, the prevalence of high LDL (≥130 mg/dL) was 25.5% (63.1 million Americans). While high total cholesterol and high LDL remain prevalent conditions in the United States, the prevalence of both conditions declined from 1999–2000 to 2017–2018. Hyperlipidemia has a substantial financial impact on U.S. health care spending; the health care cost associated with hyperlipidemia was estimated to be $26.4 billion in 2016, ranking it as the 35th most expensive health condition. Prescription pharmaceuticals and ambulatory care visits were the largest components of spending on hyperlipidemia, with contributions of 45.6% and 33.4%, respectively. The continuing growth of annual health care spending on hyperlipidemia is likely impacted by the aging U.S. population and the emergence of newer, high-cost prescription pharmaceuticals.[5] From 2017 to 2020, fewer than half of the 46.9 million adults in the U.S. who were eligible to take a statin for cholesterol management obtained a statin prescription, despite reduction in the cost of oral cholesterol-lowering medications due to the availability of generic options.[6] Medication nonadherence and suboptimal dyslipidemia control can lead to complications such as atherosclerosis, ASCVD, and death.[2]

Certain genetic conditions, comorbid metabolic conditions, medications, and patient-specific variables and behaviors are risk factors for dyslipidemia (Table 12–1).[7–9] For example, familial hypercholesteremia (FH) is a rare genetic condition characterized by high LDL levels that can be difficult to control; treatment of a patient with FH likely requires the involvement of a specialist. Poor or imbalanced diet, lack of physical activity, excessive alcohol intake, and smoking are common, controllable behaviors that contribute to lipid abnormalities. Additional patient-specific risk factors include, age, sex, race and ethnicity, and family history.[10] HCPs should perform a comprehensive patient evaluation to identify and address secondary causes of dyslipidemia and evaluate the patient's risk for ASCVD. In addition to evaluating objective cholesterol levels,

HCPs should use the ASCVD Risk Estimator Plus to estimate a patient's 10-year ASCVD risk for primary prevention.[2] The Risk Estimator uses a validated pooled cohort equation (PCE) to support clinician-patient risk discussion and optimize treatment decisions.[11] It evaluates other risk factors for ASCVD, including current age, sex, race, cigarette smoking, blood pressure, and presence of diabetes.[2,12]

Table 12–1. Secondary causes of dyslipidemia

Common conditions	Common medications
Acute hepatitis	Anticonvulsants
Diabetes	Antipsychotics (second generation > first generation)
Chronic renal failure	Beta blockers
Hypothyroidism	Corticosteroids
Malnutrition	Diuretics (thiazide > loop)
Obesity	Estrogens and progestins
Obstructive liver disease	Retinoids
Pregnancy	Sodium-glucose co-transporter 2 (SGLT-2) inhibitors

Many cholesterol-lowering medications require monitoring of liver function. Aspartate aminotransferase (AST) and alanine aminotransferase (ALT) are intracellular enzymes referred to collectively as aminotransferases, or more concisely, transaminases, which are involved in protein metabolism and gluconeogenesis. While transaminases are often included in laboratory test panels referred to as liver function tests (LFTs), their presence in the serum simply indicates tissue damage and levels are not indicative of actual liver function.

ALT is primarily found in the liver. In addition to its presence in the liver, AST is found in cardiac muscle, skeletal muscle, kidney, and pancreatic tissues at concentrations higher than those of ALT. The presence of AST or ALT in serum is indicative of tissue injury, with ALT being more specific for the liver than AST. Elevations in serum AST and ALT occur early in liver injury and are often present prior to clinical symptoms such as abdominal pain, dark-colored urine, jaundice, unusual fatigue or weakness, loss of appetite, nausea and vomiting, and pruritus. There are both hepatic and non-hepatic etiologies for elevations in serum transaminase levels, which limits their utility for evaluation of hepatoxicity without other tests.[13]

Clinical Presentation of Dyslipidemia

Patients who present with dyslipidemia are often asymptomatic. The American College of Cardiology (ACC) and American Heart Association (AHA) Task Force on Clinical Practice Guidelines recommends that all adults 20 years and older complete screening for dyslipidemia every 4 to 6 years.[2] Patients may be screened earlier or more frequently if additional risk factors or enhancers are present. Screening should include a lipid panel and risk assessment.

Untreated or uncontrolled dyslipidemia may lead to acute or chronic complications. Chronic complications of dyslipidemia include fatal and nonfatal ASCVD events. Clinical ASCVD is defined as acute coronary syndrome (ACS), history of myocardial infarction (MI), stable or unstable angina or coronary or other arterial revascularization, stroke, transient ischemic attack (TIA), or peripheral artery disease (PAD), including aortic aneurysm.[2] Secondary to hypertriglyceridemia, patients may present with acute pancreatitis and experience clinical symptoms, such as severe abdominal pain, tachycardia, nausea and vomiting, and fever.

Diagnosis

Lipid Abnormalities

A lipid panel directly measures total cholesterol, HDL, and triglycerides. LDL is calculated using the Friedewald equation [(LDL) = (Total Cholesterol) − (HDL) − (Triglycerides/5)] because direct measurement is difficult and would require ultracentrifugation.[14] The Friedewald equation is a validated tool, but it may produce erroneous results when LDL levels are low (<70 mg/dL) or triglyceride levels are high. A fasting or nonfasting lipid panel is used for diagnosis of dyslipidemia in patients aged 20 years and older. Fasting or nonfasting results are appropriate to use for the Risk Estimator to determine if pharmacotherapy is appropriate. Patients who have consumed a high-fat meal in the past eight hours should repeat their lipid panel on another occasion. If a nonfasting panel yields results indicative of hypertriglyceridemia (≥400 mg/dL), the profile should be repeated in a fasting state.[2]

The optimal ranges of lipid panel results may vary among clinical practice guidelines. Most providers follow the diagnostic criteria included in Table 12-2 for dyslipidemia and emphasize elevated LDL as the primary target for pharmacotherapy.[2,7,15] Patients may be diagnosed with dyslipidemia if their total cholesterol, triglycerides, or LDL are above optimal ranges or if their HDL is low.

Table 12-2. Diagnostic criteria for dyslipidemia

Lipid panel (mg/dL)		Low	Optimal	Borderline high	High	Very high
Total cholesterol			<200	200–239	≥240	
Triglycerides			<150	150–199	200–499	≥500
HDL	Men	<40	≥60[a]			
	Women	<50				
LDL			<100[b]; <130[c]	130–159	160–189	≥190

[a]HCPs may target a goal of ≥40 (men) or ≥50 (women).
[b]The optimal LDL range or goal may vary among clinical practice guidelines and professional organizations.
[c]An LDL range of 100–129 mg/dL is considered near optimal.

Liver Abnormalities

The common reference ranges for AST and ALT are both approximately 0 to 35 units/L. Laboratories and POCT devices typically establish specific reference ranges based on patient population variables, such as sex or BMI, or the assay technique utilized. These specific reference ranges should be utilized when available. The high end of each of these ranges is referred to as the upper limit of normal (ULN). Transaminase levels that are persistently >3 times the ULN warrant further evaluation.[16]

Physical Assessment

There is no required physical assessment to evaluate a patient for dyslipidemia. Patients may have other comorbid metabolic conditions that require physical assessment, such as hypertension, diabetes, or obesity.

Point-of-Care Testing

Lipid panel testing may be conducted as a blood test in a laboratory setting or with a POCT device in a non-laboratory setting. Lipid panel testing may be used for screening, diagnosis, and monitoring of conditions or medications. Liver function testing may be used to determine the appropriateness of pharmacotherapy and monitor adverse effects. To incorporate POCTs, HCPs should choose a CLIA-waived device and ensure that their practice meets all CLIA requirements for testing.

Lipid panel POCTs offer several advantages over laboratory-based tests as they are more accessible and produce quick results, often within 5 minutes or less. Available tests use an enzymatic reaction to produce a color change, reflectance photometry to measure light intensity, or electrochemical technology to measure an electric current to produce results. More complex devices, such as the Piccolo Xpress, may use centrifugation. Tests require a fingerstick to collect a small (40–100 μL) capillary whole-blood sample. Manufacturers recommend that HCPs wipe away the first drop of blood to improve accuracy, as it could contain tissue fluid, which may contaminate the sample and lead to inaccurate results. The requirement for phlebotomy training to collect venous whole-blood samples limits the utility of tests requiring such samples in non-laboratory settings.

Numerous CLIA-waived POCTs are available for HCPs to use in practice (Table 12–3).[17] The CardioChek Plus Analyzer and Cholestech LDX Analyzer are the most commonly used devices for cholesterol monitoring.[18–20] These devices are relatively affordable and produce results relatively quickly. In comparison with these devices, the Piccolo Xpress can analyze a wider range of blood chemistry tests, including lipid panels and transaminases, but its use for the sole purpose of cholesterol monitoring is limited by its cost.[21] While each of the devices mentioned above has advantages and disadvantages, each device meets the National Cholesterol Education Program guidelines for accuracy and precision and is certified by the Cholesterol Reference Method Laboratory Network (CRMLN) standards program of the CDC. Additional POCTs for lipid testing include the Accutrend Plus System, AimStrip Tandem Lipid Measuring System, CURO L5 Cholesterol Test Kit, CURO L7 Cholesterol Test Kit, FORA 6 Cholesterol Test Kit, LipidoCare Analyzer, LipidPro Analyzer, and Mission Cholesterol System.[17] The intended use, analytes measured, portability, storage requirements, and cost of these tests vary. Before selecting a POCT, HCPs should determine whether it is intended for HCP use or at-home use.

The Piccolo Xpress is the only CLIA-waived POCT analyzer that is currently available for monitoring of AST and ALT. The SPOTCHEM™ EZ SP-4430 previously offered lipid and liver transaminase monitoring, but the device has since been discontinued in the United States.[22] Due to the relatively high cost and limited availability of POCT analyzers for transaminase monitoring, HCPs who wish to initiate statin therapy for a patient may need to order a laboratory blood draw for be tested for transaminases prior to statin initiation or contact another provider associated with the patient's care to determine whether the patient's serum transaminase levels have been assessed recently.

Table 12-3. Lipid panel and liver function POCTs

Analyzer device	Testing details	Estimated cost[a]	Notes
CardioChek Plus (PTS Diagnostics) https://ptsdiagnostics.com/ cardiochek-plus-analyzer/	Lipid Panel (TC, HDL, TRIG, LDL[b], nHDL[b], LDL/HDL[b], TC/HDL[b]) Lipid Panel + eGLU Bundle (TC, HDL, TRIG, LDL[b], nHDL[b], LDL/HDL[b], TC/HDL[b], GLU)	Device: $1,400 Lipid Panel strips: $200/15 tests Lipid Panel + eGLU Bundle strips: $200/15 tests	Result time: 90 seconds Number of CLIA-waived analytes: 4 Reference intervals • TC: 100 to 400 mg/dL • HDL: 15 to 100 mg/dL • TG: 50 to 500 mg/dL • GLU: 40 to 600 mg/dL Other: • Battery-powered • Test strips stored at room temperature • Lot-specific MEMo chip for calibration • Fingerstick blood sample
Cholestech LDX (Abbott/Alere) https://www.global-pointofcare.abbott/en/product-details/cholestech-ldx-system.html	Lipid Panel (TC, HDL, TRIG, LDL[b], nHDL[b], TC/HDL[ba]) Lipid Panel + GLU (TC, HDL, TRIG, LDL[b], nHDL[b], TC/HDL[b], GLU)	Device: $2,800 Lipid Panel cassettes: $150/10 tests Lipid Panel +GLU cassettes: $165/10 tests	Result time: 5 minutes Number of CLIA-waived analytes: 4 Reference intervals • TC: 100 to 500 mg/dL • HDL: 15 to 100 mg/dL • TG: 45 to 650 mg/dL • GLU: 50 to 500 mg/dL Other: • Requires wall outlet for power; option to purchase battery pack • Device stored at room temperature; cassettes require refrigeration • Fingerstick blood sample

Table 12-3 cont'd

Piccolo Xpress (Abbott/Abaxis) https://www.global-pointofcare.abbott/en/product-details/apoc/piccolo-xpress-chemistry-analyzer.html	Lipid Panel (TC, HDL, TRIG, LDL[b], nHDL[b], VLDL[b], TC/HDL[b]) Lipid Panel Plus (TC, HDL, TRIG, LDL[b], nHDL[b], VLDL[b], TC/HDL[b], AST, ALT, GLU)	Device: $23,000 Lipid Panel disks: $130/10 pack Lipid Panel Plus disks: $160/10 pack	Result time: 12 minutes Number of CLIA-waived analytes: 18 Reference intervals • ALT: 10 to 47 units/L • AST: 11 to 38 units/L • TC: 20 to 520 mg/dL • HDL: 15 to 100 mg/dL • TG: 20 to 500 mg/dL Other: • Requires wall outlet for power • Device stored at room temperature; disks require refrigeration • Fingerstick blood sample for Lipid Panel and Lipid Panel Plus; others require whole-blood sample via venipuncture

[a]Pricing was estimated from an online supplier (accessed May 7, 2023).
[b]Values calculated.

Interferences

For accurate results, HCPs should ensure they review test lot and expiration dates and perform routine quality control procedures. Device manufacturers provide information on situations and substances that may interfere with tests and produce inaccurate or incomplete results. Testing interferences vary by manufacturer, but may include excessive squeezing of the finger, incomplete samples, or delays in sample collection or sample dispensing. Some POCT devices may be impacted by extremely high doses of ascorbic acid (vitamin C), abnormal hematocrit levels, strenuous exercise, use of topical cosmetics with glycerol at the testing site, and use of medications such as dopamine or methyldopa. Glycerol in hand creams, lotions, or soaps may falsely elevate triglyceride levels. Therefore, HCPs should avoid touching the sample collection pipette to the patient's skin. For levels that are unable to be measured per manufacturer reference intervals, HCPs should refer patients for laboratory testing. If HCPs suspect erroneous results, they should reference the device manual and may consider repeat testing or medical referral.

Treatment of Dyslipidemia

Treatment Goals

The goals of lipid POCT are (1) screening and early detection of dyslipidemia or ASCVD risk factors, (2) initiating and optimizing cholesterol-lowering medications, and (3) monitoring of dyslipidemia control and response to medications.

General Treatment Approach

HCPs may utilize various clinical practice guidelines including, but not limited to, the ACC/AHA,[2] American Diabetes Association (ADA),[23] and National Lipid Association (NLA).[24] HCP scope will vary based on practice design and provider capabilities. In outpatient, community-based settings, HCPs may incorporate POCT for lipids for health and wellness services or in accordance with a state-specific protocol, standing order, or agreement. The scope of practice and criteria vary by state, and pharmacists should contact their state board of pharmacy for current state-specific information. Some states permit pharmacists to initiate statin therapy. For example, pharmacists in Colorado may prescribe statin therapy in compliance with a structured statewide collaborative pharmacy protocol. Pharmacists follow a detailed algorithm with specified clinical practice guidelines, evaluate inclusion and exclusion criteria, select medication therapy, provide comprehensive counseling, and document and communicate with the patient's PCP.[25] In Idaho, pharmacists may prescribe statins for patients with diabetes to close a gap in care defined by clinical practice guidelines. Pharmacists shall maintain a patient assessment protocol that is updated regularly, based on clinical practice guidelines and evidence-based research, and readily retrievable by the Board.[26] Washington state permits pharmacists to initiate, continue, or modify statin therapy through a collaborative drug therapy agreement with a practitioner.[27] Recently, several states have started incorporation of general language to permit pharmacist prescribing for health conditions that can be screened utilizing CLIA-waived tests, some of which require a protocol, standing order, or agreement.[28]

Nonpharmacologic Therapy

Lifestyle therapies for dyslipidemia consist of diet, exercise, weight control, and behavior changes. HCPs should recommend that patients consume a well-balanced diet and limit fat intake, with a focus on specifically limiting intake of saturated and trans fats. A well-balanced diet consists of vegetables, fruits, whole grains, low-fat proteins, and nontropical vegetable oils. For protein, patients should incorporate low-fat dairy and poultry products, fish, and nuts, while limiting the consumption of red and processed meats. Patients should also limit alcohol intake (≤2 drink per day for men and ≤1 drink per day for women) and quit smoking. Making changes in dietary composition while engaging in consistent aerobic physical activity (3–5 times per week for 90–150 minutes total) can effectively contribute to weight control and facilitate weight loss. In patients who are overweight or obese, caloric intake monitoring and caloric deficits can lead to sustained, healthy weight loss, thereby lowering cholesterol levels and reducing the risk of ASCVD.[2,12]

Pharmacologic Therapy

The pharmacologic treatment of dyslipidemia may vary based on the patient's lipid panel and resulting abnormality. However, statins continue to be the mainstay of treatment, because reducing LDL remains the primary target for pharmacotherapy for ASCVD risk reduction. Additionally, current state-specific protocols, standing orders, or agreements for initiation of cholesterol-lowering medications almost exclusively permit statin prescribing only. Statins are categorized by their intensity and expected LDL lowering effect (low-intensity, <30%; moderate-intensity, 30–49%; high-intensity, ≥50%). HCPs should evaluate a patient's baseline lipid panel, liver function, current medications, and indications for referral. Prior to initiating medications, HCPs should evaluate baseline AST and ALT.[2,29] Several statins require renal dose adjustments; therefore, HCPs may find it prudent to evaluate renal function prior to initiation or select a statin that does not require renal dose adjustment.[2] HCPs may perform this evaluation by ordering tests directly, consulting the patient's provider, or accessing the patient's electronic or printed health records. If appropriate, HCPs should follow current clinical practice guidelines to initiate a statin of appropriate intensity that does not interact with the patient's current medications (Figure 1).[2,23,24] Patients with other lipid abnormalities, such as hypertriglyceridemia or severely elevated levels, meet criteria for medical referral, because other cholesterol-lowering medications or interventions may be more appropriate. Additional common, nonstatin medications include cholesterol absorption inhibitors, fibrates, omega-3 fatty acids, bile acid sequestrants, proprotein convertase subtilisin/kexin type 9 (PCSK9) inhibitors, niacin or nicotinic acid, and adenosine triphosphate-citrate lyase (ACL) inhibitors.

Figure 12–1. Statin Treatment Initiation Algorithm

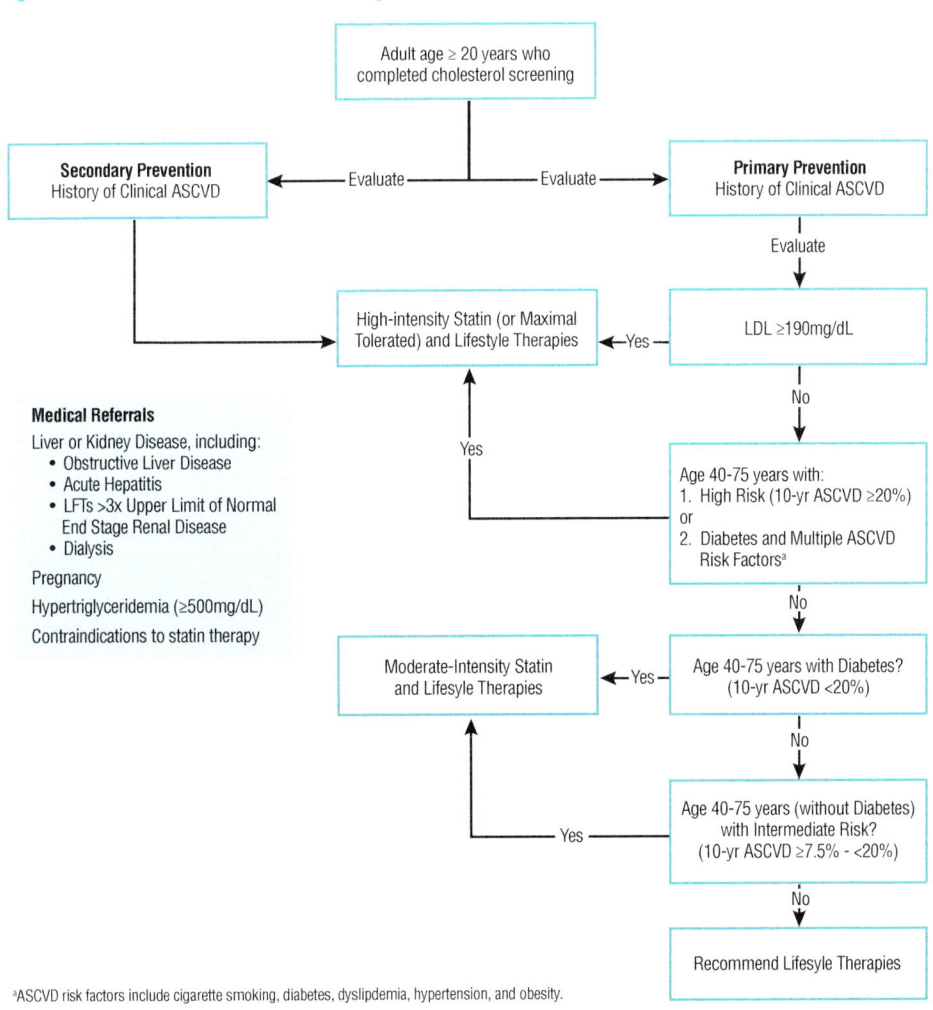

[a]ASCVD risk factors include cigarette smoking, diabetes, dyslipdemia, hypertension, and obesity.

Following initiation of statin therapy, HCPs should perform monitoring for safety and efficacy (Table 12-4). Routine periodic monitoring of transaminases in all patients on statin therapy is not recommended, because it may identify those with isolated increased AST or ALT levels, which could persuade providers to discontinue statin therapy, thus placing these patients at increased risk for cardiovascular events. Patients with increased ASCVD risk and underlying chronic, stable liver disease should be monitored closely; however, statin therapy is not contraindicated in this population. Patients with a persistent increase (remains elevated with repeat testing) in AST or ALT of >3 times the ULN should have their statin dose reduced or discontinued.[2] Active liver disease or unexplained persistent AST or ALT elevations are contraindications to statin therapy.[30,31] Patients with a baseline AST or ALT >3 times the ULN should be referred to their PCP for further evaluation.

While statins are widely used and well tolerated in many individuals, patients may experience statin-associated adverse effects. The most common adverse effect of statins is muscle pain or myalgia. Certain factors may predispose a patient to experience adverse effects as a result of statin use, including age, female sex, low BMI, Asian ancestry, excess alcohol intake, and certain medications and comorbidities. If patients experience myalgia, HCPs may reduce the dose or rechallenge with an alternate statin. More serious, but rare, adverse effects include rhabdomyolysis, hepatic failure, transaminase elevation, new-onset diabetes, and impaired memory. HCPs may opt to monitor creatinine kinase (CK) levels at baseline or in patients who are experiencing severe muscle aches and pains as a screening measure for rhabdomyolysis, which can be life-threatening or result in permanent disability.

Approximately 1% to 2% of patients on statin therapy experience asymptomatic, reversible transaminase elevations.[13] These transient increases in transaminase levels generally occur in the first few months of statin therapy. Asymptomatic increases in levels of transaminases to >3 times the ULN are infrequently associated with statin therapy and often resolve with dose reduction or use of an alternative statin. A thorough evaluation for nonstatin etiologies is warranted when significant transaminase elevations persist. Serious hepatotoxicity with statin therapy is rare and likely idiosyncratic in nature.[2]

Table 12-4. Laboratory monitoring parameters

Test	Recommended frequency	Notes
Lipid panel (fasting preferred)	At baseline, 4-12 weeks after statin initiation or dose adjustment, then every 3-12 months thereafter.	Screen all adults 20 years and older every 4 to 6 years; screen more frequently if risk factors are present.
Transaminases (AST and ALT)	At baseline, then only if symptoms suggesting hepatoxicity develop.	Routine measurements are not recommended.
Creatinine kinase (CK)	Only if severe statin-associated muscle symptoms or objective muscle weakness develop.	CLIA-waved tests for CK are not available. Referral required.

Indications for Referral

Referral to a PCP may be warranted prior to initiating statin therapy or during statin therapy. Reasons for medical referral prior to initiating statin therapy are included in Figure 12–1.

Referral to a PCP may be necessary if issues related to efficacy or adverse effects are identified during statin therapy. Patients with suboptimal responses to maximally tolerated statin regimens should be referred to determine whether additional, nonstatin therapies are warranted. Patients who develop statin-associated adverse effects such as persistently elevated transaminases or severe, unresolved muscle aches and pains should also be referred for further evaluation.

Patient Cases

Patient Case 12–1 SOAP Note

Collect	Chief complaint
Subjective	MH, a 43-year-old Black male, presents for a biometric health screening.
	History of present illness (HPI)
	He reports no general concerns except his father recently had a stroke and he wants to make sure he is maintaining a healthy lifestyle.
Objective	Past medical history (PMH): hypertension (4 years), atrial fibrillation (2 years)
	Family history (FH): Mother is 66 years old with hypertension and type 2 diabetes mellitus. Father is 68 years old with recent ischemic stroke, hypertension, and hyperlipidemia. No siblings.
	Social history (SH): Smokes cigarettes (1 pack per day for 20 years), consumes 1 to 2 cans of beer (8-ounce) most evenings. Denies recreational substance use.
	Medication list: amlodipine 10 mg once daily (4 years) metoprolol succinate 100 mg once daily (2 years) rivaroxaban 20 mg once daily (2 years) famotidine 10 mg twice daily as needed (10 years) ibuprofen 200 to 400 mg every 8 hours as needed (20 years)
	Allergies: lisinopril (angioedema)
	Review of symptoms (ROS): non-contributory
	BP: 134/86 mm Hg Pulse: 68 bpm Height: 74 in Weight: 210 lbs
	Today, Lipid Panel + Glu per Cholestech LDX™ (fasting): TC: 178 mg/dL GLU: 142 mg/dL HDL: 40 mg/dL LDL: 109 mg/dL TRIG: 144 mg/dL

Patient Case 12–1 SOAP Note cont'd

Assess	Since this patient does not have a history of clinical ASCVD, we need to determine if he is considered high risk for ASCVD.
	General risk factors include cigarette smoking, diabetes, dyslipidemia, hypertension, and obesity. This patient smokes cigarettes and is receiving treatment for hypertension. Based on his lipid panel, he does not currently have dyslipidemia. His body mass index (BMI) is 27, which categorizes him as overweight, but not obese.
	To make a more informed decision as to whether statin therapy is recommended, his 10-year ASCVD risk should be calculated. Based on the ASCVD Risk Estimator Plus, his 10-year ASCVD risk is 11.6%, placing him at an intermediate risk level. Based on these results, he could benefit from moderate-intensity statin therapy.
Plan	Prior to initiating moderate-intensity statin therapy, baseline liver enzymes should be assessed. Since the Cholestech LDX™ does not offer measurement of AST and ALT, the patient's PCP should be contacted to obtain recent values or to order the tests for completion at a laboratory. Smoking cessation lifestyle changes should also be recommended.
Implement	Contact the patient's PCP to obtain and evaluate liver enzymes. If appropriate, recommend initiating a moderate-intensity statin.
Monitor/ Follow-up	After initiating statin therapy, a fasting lipid panel should be reassessed in 4 to 12 weeks and then every 3 to 12 months thereafter. Liver transaminase testing is required only if the patient develops signs or symptoms suggestive of hepatoxicity.

Patient Case 12–2 SOAP Note

Collect	Chief complaint
Subjective	CT, a 56-year-old Asian female, presents for her first follow-up lipid panel appointment.
	HPI
	She initiated statin therapy 6 weeks ago. Since then, she has also self-initiated a red yeast rice dietary supplement, reduced her intake of foods containing saturated fat, and increased her activity level by walking for 30 minutes 3 times per week instead of just once or twice weekly.
Objective	PMH: hyperlipidemia (6 weeks), hypertension (8 years), type 2 diabetes mellitus (5 years), seasonal allergies (15 years), and bilateral knee osteoarthritis (1 year) FH: Mother is 81 years old with hypertension and osteoporosis. Father deceased at age 63 due to myocardial infarction; his medical conditions included type 2 diabetes mellitus, hypertension, and hyperlipidemia. No siblings.
	SH: Denies use of tobacco products, drinks 1–2 glasses of wine (4-ounce) most evenings. Denies recreational substance use.
	Medication list: atorvastatin 40 mg once daily (6 weeks) empagliflozin 10 mg once daily (2 years) hydrochlorothiazide 25 mg once daily (2 years) lisinopril 40 mg once daily (6 years) metformin 1,000 mg twice daily (5 years) acetaminophen 500 to 1,000 mg 3 times per day (1 year) diclofenac sodium 1% topical gel 4 grams to knees 4 times per day (3 months) levocetirizine 5 mg once daily (2 years) glucosamine 1500 mg/chondroitin 800 mg complex twice daily (3 months) red yeast rice 600 mg twice daily (4 weeks)

Patient Case 12-2 SOAP Note cont'd

	Allergies: NKDA
	ROS: Denies muscle pain or dark-colored urine. No discoloration to eyes or skin noted.
	BP: 132/84 mm Hg Pulse: 74 bpm Height: 68 in Weight: 170 lb
	Today, Lipid Panel Plus per Piccolo Xpress (fasting): ALT: 320 units/L, AST: 245 units/L, TC: 185 mg/dL, GLU: 128 mg/dL, HDL: 45 mg/dL, LDL: 116 mg/dL, TRIG: 119 mg/dL
	Baseline 6 weeks ago, Lipid Panel Plus per Piccolo Xpress (fasting): ALT: 20 units/L, AST: 15 units/L, TC: 240 mg/dL, GLU: 130 mg/dL, HDL: 35 mg/dL, LDL: 171 mg/dL, TRIG: 170 mg/dL
Assess	While the patient's total and LDL cholesterol levels are trending down and her HDL level is trending up nicely with atorvastatin therapy, her AST and ALT levels are greater than three times the ULN. The patient self-initiated red yeast rice therapy (initiated since her last visit) and the use of red yeast rice concurrently with statins should be avoided, because it may increase her risk of statin-associated adverse effects such as myopathy and liver dysfunction. Her increase in knee pain is likely due to a recent increase in physical activity.
Plan	Instruct the patient to discontinue the red yeast rice dietary supplement. While her serum transaminase elevations may be due to the interaction between the red yeast rice and atorvastatin, the patient should be referred to her PCP for further evaluation because her transaminase levels are >3 times the ULN.
Implement	Refer the patient to her PCP. Recommend discontinuing red yeast rice dietary supplement. Monitor liver enzymes.
Monitor/ Follow-up	If her serum transaminase elevations persist despite discontinuation of the red yeast rice and other etiologies are not determined, she may be experiencing statin-induced liver damage, which would warrant either a statin dose reduction or discontinuation of statin therapy.

References

1. Centers for Disease Control and Prevention. About Cholesterol. Atlanta, GA: CDC. Available at: https://www.cdc.gov/cholesterol/about.htm. Accessed May 1, 2023.

2. Grundy SM, Stone NJ, Bailey AL, et al. 2018 AHA/ACC/AACVPR/AAPA/ABC/ACPM/ADA/AGS/APhA/ASPC/NLA/PCNA guideline on the management of blood cholesterol: executive summary: A report of the American College of Cardiology/American Heart Association Task Force on Clinical Practice Guidelines. *Circulation.* 2019;139:e1046–e1081. doi:10.1161/CIR.0000000000000624

3. American Heart Association. HDL (Good), LDL (Bad) Cholesterol and Triglycerides. Dallas, TX: AHA. Available at: https://www.heart.org/en/health-topics/cholesterol/hdl-good-ldl-bad-cholesterol-and-triglycerides. Accessed May 1, 2023.

4. American Heart Association. What is Atherosclerosis? Dallas, TX: AHA. Available at: https://www.heart.org/en/health-topics/cholesterol/about-cholesterol/atherosclerosis. Accessed May 1, 2023.

5. Tsao CW, Aday AW, Almarzooq ZI, et al. Heart disease and stroke statistics—2023 update: a report from the American Heart Association. *Circulation.* 2023;147(8):e93–e621. doi:10.1161/CIR.0000000000001123

6. Wall HK, Ritchey MD, Gillespie C, et al. Vital Signs: Prevalence of key cardiovascular disease risk factors for Million Hearts 2022—United States, 2011–2016. *MMWR Morb Mortal Wkly Rep.* 2018;67(35):983–991. doi:10.15585/mmwr.mm6735a4

7. Expert Panel on Detection, Evaluation, and Treatment of High Blood Cholesterol in Adults. Executive Summary of the Third Report of the National Cholesterol Education Program (NCEP) Expert Panel on Detection, Evaluation, and Treatment of High Blood Cholesterol in Adults (Adult Treatment Panel III). *JAMA.* 2001;285(19):2486–2497. doi:10.1001/jama.285.19.2486

8. Vodnala D, Rubenfire M, Brook RD. Secondary causes of dyslipidemia. *Am J Cardiol.* 2012;110(6):823–825. doi:10.1016/j.amjcard.2012.04.062

9. Henkin Y, Como JA, Oberman A. Secondary dyslipidemia. Inadvertent effects of drugs in clinical practice. *JAMA.* 1992;267(7):961–968. doi:10.1001/jama.267.7.961

10. Centers for Disease Control and Prevention. Know Your Risk for High Cholesterol. Atlanta, GA: CDC. Available at: https://www.cdc.gov/cholesterol/risk_factors.htm. Accessed May 1, 2023.

11. Martin SS, Sperling LS, Blaha MJ, et al. Clinician-patient risk discussion for atherosclerotic cardiovascular disease prevention. *J Am Coll Cardiol.* 2015;65:1361–8. doi:10.1016/j.jacc.2015.01.043

12. American College of Cardiology. ASCVD Risk Estimator Plus. Washington, DC: ACC. Available at: https://tools.acc.org/ascvd-risk-estimator-plus/#!/calculate/estimate/. Accessed May 19, 2023.

13. Bethea ED, Pratt DS. Evaluation of Liver Function. In: Loscalzo J, Fauci A, Kasper D, Hauser S, Longo D, Jameson J. eds. *Harrison's Principles of Internal Medicine, 21e.* McGraw Hill; 2022.

14. Friedewald WT, Levy RI, Fredrickson DS. Estimation of the concentration of low-density lipoprotein cholesterol in plasma, without use of the preparative ultracentrifuge. *Clin Chem.* 1972;18(6):499–502. doi:10.1093/clinchem/18.6.499

15. Arnett DK, Blumenthal RS, Albert MA, et al. 2019 ACC/AHA guideline on the primary prevention of cardiovascular disease: a report of the American College of Cardiology/American Heart Association Task Force on Clinical Practice Guidelines. *Circulation.* 2019;140:e596–e646. doi:10.1161/CIR.0000000000000678

16. Nicoll D, Mark Lu C, McPhee SJ. Lab Tests. In: Nicoll D, Mark Lu C, McPhee SJ, eds. *Guide to Diagnostic Tests, 7e.* McGraw Hill; 2017.

17. U.S. Food and Drug Administration. CLIA-Clinical Laboratory Improvement Amendments. Silver Spring, MD: FDA. Available at: https://www.accessdata.fda.gov/scripts/cdrh/cfdocs/cfCLIA/search.cfm. Accessed May 17, 2023.

18. PTS Diagnostics. CardioChek Plus Analyzer. Available at: https://ptsdiagnostics.com/cardiochek-plus-analyzer/. Accessed May 8, 2023.

19. Alere, San Deigo, Inc. Cholestech LDX Analyzer. Available at: https://www.globalpointofcare.abbott/en/product-details/cholestech-ldx-system.html. Accessed May 12, 2023.

20. Haggerty L, Tran D. Cholesterol point-of-care testing for community pharmacies: A review of the current literature. *J Pharm Pract.* 2017 Aug;30(4):451–458. doi:10.1177/0897190016645023

21. Abaxis. Piccolo Xpress Analyzer. Available at: https://www.globalpointofcare.abbott/en/product-details/apoc/piccolo-xpress-chemistry-analyzer.html. Accessed May 12, 2023.

22. ARKRAY USA, Inc. SPOTCHEM™ EZ Chemistry Analyzer. Available at: https://www.arkrayusa.com/english/clinical_diagnostics/products/dry_chemistry/spotchem_ez_sp-4430.html. Accessed May 22, 2023.

23. ElSayed NA, Aleppo G, Aroda VR, et al. Cardiovascular disease and risk management: Standards of Care in Diabetes—2023. *Diabetes Care.* 2023;46(Suppl. 1):S158–S190. doi:10.2337/dc23-S010

24. National Lipid Association (NLA). 2018 Guideline on the management of blood cholesterol – NLA perspective. Available at: https://www.lipid.org/2018-guidelines-nla-perspective. Accessed May 19, 2023.
25. Colorado State Board of Pharmacy. Collaborative Pharmacy Practice & Statewide Protocols. Available at: https://dpo.colorado.gov/Pharmacy/Protocols. Accessed May 17, 2023.
26. Idaho Board of Pharmacy. Law book with Idaho pharmacy code & administrative rules. Available at: https://adminrules.idaho.gov/rules/2018%20Archive/27/270104.pdf. Accessed May 17, 2023.
27. Washington Board of Pharmacy. Guidance on Collaborative Drug Therapy Agreements. Available at: https://doh.wa.gov/sites/default/files/legacy/Documents/Pubs/690327.pdf. Accessed May 22, 2023.
28. National Alliance of State Pharmacy Associations. Pharmacist Prescribing: "Test and Treat." Richmond, VA: NASPA. Available at: https://naspa.us/resource/pharmacist-prescribing-for-strep-and-flu-test-and-treat/. Accessed May 17, 2023.
29. U.S. Food and Drug Administration. FDA Drug Safety Communication: Important safety label changes to cholesterol-lowering statin drugs [press announcement]. Silver Spring, MD: FDA. Available at: https://www.fda.gov/drugs/drug-safety-and-availability/fda-drug-safety-communication-important-safety-label-changes-cholesterol-lowering-statin-drugs. Accessed May 20, 2023.
30. Lipitor [product information]. New York, NY: Pfizer; 2022.
31. Zocor [product information]. Jersey City, NJ: Organon Pharma; 2022.